Handbook of
Adolescent Medicine and Health Promotion

Handbook of
Adolescent Medicine
and Health Promotion

David MN Paperny, MD, FAAP, FSAHM

University of Hawaii, USA

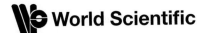 **World Scientific**

NEW JERSEY · LONDON · SINGAPORE · BEIJING · SHANGHAI · HONG KONG · TAIPEI · CHENNAI

Published by

World Scientific Publishing Co. Pte. Ltd.

5 Toh Tuck Link, Singapore 596224

USA office: 27 Warren Street, Suite 401-402, Hackensack, NJ 07601

UK office: 57 Shelton Street, Covent Garden, London WC2H 9HE

British Library Cataloguing-in-Publication Data
A catalogue record for this book is available from the British Library.

HANDBOOK OF ADOLESCENT MEDICINE AND HEALTH PROMOTION

ISBN-13 978-981-4317-98-6
ISBN-10 981-4317-98-5

Typeset by Stallion Press
Email: enquiries@stallionpress.com

Printed by FuIsland Offset Printing (S) Pte Ltd. Singapore

To my son, Jerry,
who taught me the most about adolescence,
and how to really walk the walk and talk the talk!

Preface

Because of new adolescent and young adult health and societal issues, *medical diseases* are no longer the main health threats to their well-being. We must preempt and respond to the consequences of *behavioral choices* faced by more and more adolescents worldwide, such as the complications of unintended pregnancy, STDs including HIV, alcohol and drug abuse, and emotional issues including suicide and eating disorders. There is the risk of future heart disease related to smoking, exercise behaviors, and nutrition, as well as the negative consequences of so many accidental injuries, particularly those related to motor vehicle accidents. This ongoing health crisis requires a fundamental change in the emphasis of adolescent health services — to services which are directed at the *prevention* of the major health threats facing today's youth. This handbook, therefore, focuses on such services, as well as uniquely-adolescent aspects of medical conditions, rather than detailed evaluation and management of routine medical illnesses and diseases, which can be gleaned from other medical textbooks.

The health issues of contemporary adolescents and young adults require health providers, paraprofessionals, schools, families, and communities to develop practical methods to preemptively improve the health habits and well-being of youths. Please take this handbook with you on your journey.

I would like to acknowledge and sincerely thank the following reviewers of the content of this publication:

Robert J. Bidwell MD, FAAP
Board certified in Adolescent Medicine
Associate Professor of Pediatrics
University of Hawaii, John A. Burns School of Medicine

Douglas Chun MD, FAAP, FAAD
Board certified in Pediatrics and Dermatology
Hawaii Permanente Medical Group

Warren M. Seigel MD, FAAP, FSAHM
Director Adolescent Services
Coney Island Hospital, New York

Frank Uhr MD, FAAOS, JD
Board certified Orthopedic Surgery; Fellow in Sports Medicine
Hawaii Permanente Medical Group

Adolescents are neither large children nor small adults.
David Paperny

*A bonus CD with useful resources, handouts and videos is available to book customers upon contacting the author at **DavidPaperny@aol.com***

FOREWORD

Personal histories prove that the innocence of childhood does grow into the curiosity and risk-seeking of adolescence. Parents often feel like a failure when their children do not grow into the teenager or young adult that they wanted them to be! In the past, developmentalists, or those in the health professions who have been interested in such matters, have essentially focused on the biology of change. With the availability of new imaging technologies, there has been an increased interest in correlating biology with manifest psychological development and behavior. The core determinants of change are being defined — the very determinants that brought us to our present position.

For many of us, the struggles and behaviors of today's youth are foreign. As Dr. Paperny points out in this book, these determinants of change are taking place in a different world — a different social ecology, so to speak — a world that is defined by individual communities, cultural and religious beliefs, families, school environments, recreational opportunities, access to health care, economic resources, media exposure, peer interaction and life opportunities. It is these unique social ecologies that impact the identity-seeking adolescent and influence the trajectory of his or her personal change. Hence, while the core experience of adolescence remains unchanged, the expression or adaptation to that experience differs not only from generation to generation, from community to community, but from country to country.

Simply put, the need for the journey through adolescence does not differ from yours or mine. The options for travel are different and maybe more treacherous — what we, as professionals, call *risk-taking*. Seen through their eyes, young people merely experience this risk-taking as options for their development, for their growing up, and for peer acceptance. Thus, no longer can we view adolescence as the 'healthiest period' in the life-cycle. The interface between social ecology, pubescence and psychosocial development leads to a number of diseases and disorders that challenge the traditional resources of the average health practitioner.

In a recent report on health issues in today's youth, a group of opinion leaders from American business, higher education and the military expressed a consensus concern about health issues such as obesity, poor mental health including depression, drug use, risky sexual practices and lack of resilience.[1] On the positive side, there was a general agreement that today's teens are far more knowledgeable about their health and what would help to improve it. From a business point of view, obesity led to increased risks for diabetes and hypertension, with absenteeism and increased insurance costs, while mental health issues, primarily depression and stress, lessened productivity and increased the use of short term disability, as well as family and medical leave. It was pointed out that the United States military, often the employer of last resort for at-risk youth, now refuses entry to over half of the youth recruits due to health issues. A recent study from the U.S. Department of Defence reported that 70% of female recruits and 62% of male recruits failed to qualify for military service because of physical or mental health conditions.[2] Opinion leaders agreed that there needs to be a new paradigm to improve the health of adolescents — one that makes a greater investment in prevention through wellness education and skills training. Like any prevention, these approaches need to go beyond the schools, health centers, family environments and recreational settings. The approaches need to create healthy lifestyles within a culture of health.

In this book, Dr. Paperny emphasizes a proactive paradigm, a paradigm of anticipatory guidance based on our knowledge of development and disease. His approach is not one which excludes our role of intervention, but one that integrates prevention into the clinical visit. He promotes a model that goes beyond culture, language and community, a model that is universal and timeless — one that makes an impact on the lives of young people not only in the present, but translates into a preventive investment in their future. It is a model that gets more 'bang for the buck' — a consideration of paramount importance in the contemporary medical marketplace.

The *Handbook of Adolescent Medicine and Health Promotion* draws on Dr. Paperny's own clinical experience as a physician working with adolescents for over 30 years. He provides practical clinical approaches that really work. He discusses approaches to comprehensive health screening and evaluation, how to impact health choices and behaviors, and integrate issues of education and health promotion. This book is a unique combination of Pediatrics, Internal Medicine, Gynecology and Psychology. It addresses the contemporary issues facing youth in this millennium, including new technology and socio-cultural matters. The emphasis is not on the subtle diagnostics and complex subspecialty concerns, nor conditions which Pediatrics or Internal Medicine routinely manages with standard clinical guidelines (that can be found in textbooks or online), but rather, "uniquely adolescent" health applications.

This handbook will be useful for health providers, residents, and health care students of all specialties involved in the clinical care of adolescents and young adults. In addition, it can be a valuable resource tool for other interdisciplinary or lay practitioners who have regular contact with youth, and who want to more effectively promote their health and well-being. Since young people are usually influenced by many paramedical specialties as well as parents, teachers and clergy, this book will be useful to the wide variety of individuals who shape their daily health choices and actions.

Within the subspecialty model of medicine, adolescent medicine may best be thought of as the geriatrics of pediatrics! Within such a model, approaches to adolescent health care must, at a bare minimum, be comprehensive, but at its best, be integrative, emphasizing behavioral, prevention and health promotion issues. This perhaps is the single most distinguishing characteristic of the practice model of adolescent medicine as compared to those of other subspecialties. This book takes up the challenge of documenting this approach by providing practical clinical information and scenarios in an easy-to-use format. If your quest is to improve health outcomes, habits of wellness and to help adolescents and young adults get the most out of life, then this Handbook is an excellent starting point!

Richard G MacKenzie MD, FAAP, FSAHM
Director (Emeritus) Division of Adolescent Medicine
Medical Director, International Programs, Children's Hospital of Los Angeles
Associate Professor Pediatrics and Medicine, University of Southern California Keck School of Medicine

References

1. Frohnen BP, McManus MA, Limb SJ, Straus CR. (2010). *Concern for Our Teens: Opinion Leaders Speak Out On Adolescent Health*. National Alliance to Advance Adolescent Health, Report Number 4, July 2010. (Washington DC).
2. Lewin Group. (2005). *Qualified Military Available: New Estimates of the Eligible Youth Population*. Prepared for Accession Policy, Office of the Under Secretary of Defense (Personnel and Readiness) (The Lewin Group, Human Resources Research Organization, Falls Church, VA).

About the Author

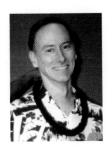

David Paperny
David Paperny, M.D. has been a Clinical Professor of Pediatrics for the John A. Burns School of Medicine at the University of Hawaii, and Director of Kaiser Permanente Adolescent Services in Hawaii for nearly 30 years. He received his medical education at University of California Los Angeles School of Medicine, completed his pediatric residency at Kapiolani-Children's Medical Center, and did his fellowship training in Adolescent Medicine at University of Washington in Seattle. He is a Fellow of the American Academy of Pediatrics and member of the Sections on Adolescent Health as well as Computers and Technology. He is a Fellow of the Society for Adolescent Health and Medicine, a certified Consultant for the Amerian Society of Clinical Hypnosis, board certified in Brainwave Biofeeedback, and a forensic medical consultant for the Hawaii Sex Abuse Treatment Center. Topics of his many publications include medical information technology, computerized health screening and assessment, as well as using computers and multimedia for health education. He has published many software programs and video-DVD programs on diverse topics such as sex education, teen parenting prevention, health assessment, asthma care skills, and parenting skills. He developed the Teen and Young Adult Checkup, a unique approach to health evaluation and education using computers, paramedical health counselors, and nurses to provide comprehensive adolescent preventive health services. His practice in Adolescent Medicine has included medical management with a focus on health education and promotion, sex education, health psychology of adolescence, biofeedback, stress management and personal empowerment.

Contents

Contents

Chapter 1

Medical and Paramedical Visits

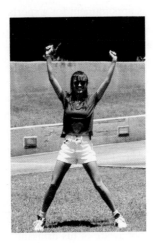

Overview

Chronic disease and early death are linked to social factors and behaviors that can be modified during adolescence and young adulthood when many health habits are formed. Many youths' health problems result from consequences of behavior choices, such as alcohol and drug use, sexual practices, physical inactivity and smoking. The common medical disease conditions, such as acne, gastroenteritis, and colds are greatly overshadowed by the impact of these social and behavioral issues.

Youths are now involved in far more serious behaviors that jeopardize their immediate and long-term health. These new contemporary problems require maximal emphasis on psychological and behavioral issues. We must use proactive prevention programs capable of reaching large numbers of youths, rather than reactive medical treatment of the results of bad health behaviors. This requires the participation of health care systems, schools, community groups, and families. Accordingly this chapter will refer to Medical and Paramedical personnel as *Health Providers*. Clinicians provide most medical services, but can also play an important role as health advocates and community leaders for improving policies and programs that affect the health of adolescents.

Consistently repeated health messages from many credible sources and various health providers that reinforce prevention are more convincing than those given to adolescents in isolation. A comprehensive health evaluation for youths should focus on the recommended areas for best overall outcomes.

A 17-year-old male kept his appointment for a sports pre-participation physical examination. The physician uses a computerized risk screening program for all health appraisals, and meets with adolescents alone before parents join them for the health evaluation. The teen's mother remained in the waiting room completing a health survey about her teen and a sports participation screening questionnaire. After the 15-minute computerized risk assessment and the clinician's review of the prioritized problem list, the private discussion with the teen confirmed moderate drinking of alcohol almost every weekend, riding monthly with friends and uncles who drive after several drinks, and the bimonthly use of marijuana. The teen patient was eager to share that he had several sexual partners with whom he never used condoms, but had no STD symptoms. He also confirmed that he had tried ice (crystal methamphetamine) several times, but had never used anabolic steroids. He was an average student who did not drive, but wanted a license. He felt his mother was somewhat aware of his drinking and that she knew he used marijuana. The mother in the waiting room was informed that the doctor was promoting health and safety through a discussion and that she would be called in soon. There was a frank discussion with the teen about riding with intoxicated drivers and alternative choices, as well as his plans to drive. The realities of ice use were shared by the office nurse who lost a son to ice use. After a 4-minute condom use video, STD screening was refused. After the physical examination, the mother was then invited into the examination room. The completed health survey and sports screening questionnaire were reviewed, and general safety issues about drugs and alcohol was discussed with both, as well as the sobering responsibilities of obtaining a driver's license. As planned, the teen requested of his mother a "No-Questions-Asked free taxi ride home safety contract." The mother signed consent for TDAP and Menactra vaccines.

Caring for Teens and Young Adults

Adolescents generally seem healthy and usually come to a medical setting for physical examinations or for an acute illness or injury. It is often said that teens are the healthiest group around, but they are vulnerable to a wide range of health problems with lasting consequences that are preventable. If recognized early, they can be managed in ways to decrease adolescent morbidity and costs of crisis care. Adolescents who come for health care do not necessarily expect to be asked about their behaviors, but if you do not ask about personal behaviors, then you are not addressing issues that put adolescents at greatest risk. Most youths do desire to discuss personal issues, but are initially uncomfortable or do not know how to express sensitive information easily. Most adolescents do want to discuss health behaviors including sexuality and substance use with their clinician. The top three desired discussion topics are drugs, sexually transmitted diseases (STD), and smoking, while the top three subjects actually addressed by providers are usually eating habits, weight, and exercise. A discussion about substance use and sexuality with youths currently engaged in these risk-taking behaviors occurs less than half the time. Since multiple studies have indicated that many adolescents feel embarrassed or are not able to initiate these discussions themselves, it is crucial that clinicians begin the conversations. Adolescents with chronic illnesses are equally engaged in risk behaviors and need to have similar discussions.

Parents also want clinicians to discuss health issues with their adolescents; 9 out of 10 parents want discussions for their teens on nutrition, substance abuse, smoking, exercise, STDs, and skin care, and 8 out of 10 consider suicide, pregnancy, contraception, safe sex, and depression to be important. Very few parents feel that these topics should not be discussed with health providers.

In the health care setting, adolescents care most about being treated respectfully as young adults — not being judged for their behavior, knowing that they are being given honest information and knowing that their personal information is kept private. For a health care provider, adolescents value certain qualities such as being friendly, caring, open, careful, respectful and experienced, as well as clean in preventing disease transmission. Although confidentiality is highly rated by adolescents, it is surpassed by knowledge, respect, honesty, and cleanliness.

What Adolescents Care Most About in the Health Care Setting
- Being treated respectfully as young adults.
- Not being judged for their behavior.
- Knowing that they are being given honest information.
- Knowing that their personal information is kept private.

Interviewing Adolescents

"We must listen before we can talk to the voice of another and even more to the voice of the heart." - Anonymous

When interviewing adolescents, each provider will tailor the approach to his or her own style. However, in order to avoid lack of full disclosure, risk-taking behaviors should not be discussed in front of the parent. The adolescent should always have an opportunity to meet with the clinician alone. Some clinicians meet with both the adolescent and parent together and then with each separately, while others meet with the adolescent first and then bring in the parent. It is helpful to also meet with the adolescent and parent together to observe the parent-adolescent interaction and facilitate communication between them.

The health interview should identify current health concerns as well as behaviors that may compromise health, so the interview should include a review of medical problems, developmental issues, as well as a health behavior history. Listen carefully and actively seek to understand precisely what the youth is trying to say. Watch for non-verbal messages that indicate discomfort, misunderstanding, or confusion. Non-verbal communication is sometimes more important than spoken words. Cues such as tone of voice, body language and posture, eye contact, facial expressions, silence, general appearance and demeanor may reflect feelings and agendas far more important to the youth than what you are asking about. Non-verbal communication is usually an accurate reflection of feelings, free of deception and distortion, and may support or contradict spoken words. If you sense a feeling, mood, or unspoken problem, comment on your observation to the youth in a caring way; this can facilitate rapport and eliminate communication obstacles.

Normally, rapport is established by initially addressing non-threatening issues, then moving to more sensitive inquiries: typical HEADSSS interview. However, the opposite is true if the provider already has rapport or has used a screening questionnaire, where, in the interest of time and priority, sensitive issues should be addressed more quickly. Ask sensitive questions permissively and some with an assumption which can be denied: "Some teens try marijuana; when was the last time you tried it?" Keep your approach non-judgmental, and offer reassurance on sensitive subjects. Use open-ended questions, and clarify things by repeating them back so the youth can verify you have interpreted them correctly. Take comments seriously so he or she feels respected, and explain or suggest things rather than lecture or moralize. Listen more than speak, and maintain a neutral attitude. Minimize note-taking, especially during sensitive discussions. Adolescents are particularly sensitive to provider attitudes and approaches, and tend to respond more emotionally rather than logically. They will appreciate the clinician who is able to minimize their fears and put them at ease.

Adolescents are highly sensitive to the examiner's tone. They may also misinterpret a suggestion of urgency as impatience or intolerance.

Respect, empathy, and a comfortable exchange of information in a shared collaborative approach are at the heart of effective interviewing. Judgmentalism, paternalism and moralizing promote distancing on the part of the youth. Teenagers are particularly appreciative of the clinician who is an authority but does not act in an authoritarian manner. Legitimacy is based on knowledge, expertise, justice, fairness, and concern. Over-identification is equally problematic. Do not confuse empathy (being sensitive to and in tune with the patient's plight) with over-identification (taking on the adolescent's problems and reacting to them as if they were your own).

Interview Principles and Techniques

Be true to your own personal style and vocabulary. The false adoption of teen jargon or mannerisms is quickly perceived as artificial and does not promote trust. Questions should be posed in clear and unambiguous terms according to the adolescent's level of cognition. Misunderstandings can lead to the conclusion that the adolescent is a poor historian, when the truth is that the questions were not framed in an appropriate or adequately concrete way. Indeed, many teenagers do want to discuss their most heartfelt concerns, provided it is with somebody they trust.

Accuracy and Depth of a Teen's Discussion About Personal Matters and Behaviors is Determined by
- The overall clinician-teen rapport.
- Concerns about the social desirability of their behavior.
- Their perception of the motive behind inquiries.
- Their perception of the clinician's personal values and biases.

Sometimes, open-ended questions such as "Tell me what's going on?" or "How long has this been a problem?" will produce only the response "I don't know." Some adolescents are simply not very verbal and "I don't know" is an easy way to cover up insecurity. Youths with very personal problems or behaviors may say "I don't know" as a way to avoid further discussion. Others are angry or depressed and simply do not want to talk. By using good open-ended questions ("What was that like...," "What do you think about that..."), the youth is in control of what to say, how to say it, and how much to say. The provider finds out what the youth wants to emphasize, and it gives responsibility for the discussion to him or her. Leading, yet permissive questions can direct the discussion ("Some people have done that. When was the last time you did it?"). The hypothetical question is useful ("If someone was really upset at his friend..."). Sometimes, a choice question is needed ("When some people say that, they mean A or B. Which do you mean?"). Remember to address the adolescent's agenda, not only yours or the parent's (e.g. "What are the things you worry about the most?").

Interview Techniques Dos & Don'ts

Do:
- Clarify — ("What do you mean?")
- Encourage — ("Tell me more.")
- Interpret — ("Do you think that you're feeling that your friend doesn't trust you?")
- Reflect — ("It really hurt you.")
- Use a genuine tone of voice and good eye contact.
- Be responsive and flexible.
- Express honest concern — ("I am worried that if you don't use condoms you may…)
- Sense the feelings — ("I guess you really don't want to be here…").
- Be honest — ("Your mom told my nurse that you are…").

Do not:
- Give quick advice — ("Why don't you just…").
- Don't moralize or give your own opinions — ("You really should…").
- Never criticize or put down — ("That's really not...").
- Don't judge — ("That's terribly...").

A number of structured interviewing techniques can be helpful to elicit information from adolescents:

- Numerical rating scale
  Patients who have problems describing the severity of their problem may be able to use a numerical rating scale: "On a scale of 1 to 5, how bad is your family situation?" Always define your scale — explain 5 is worst in this case.
- Mini-Likert scale
  The use of an abbreviated Likert scale can also elicit useful information through questions such as "Do you feel about the same, more troubled or less troubled about… (your school performance) than your friends?"
- Change wishes
  The adolescent is asked if there are any changes about the situation that would help: "If there was one thing you could change to make the situation better, what would it be?", or "If you could change yourself, your family, your life… (etc.), what

two things would you like to change and how?" This inquiry gives insight into the patient's level of cognitive maturation.

- Indirection end projection
  The patient's views about the behavior in general or asking about the behavior of friends: "Do any of your friends smoke?", "What do people in your school think about...?", and "Are any of your friends involved in...?" As adolescents tend to project their own experiences when answering, responses often suggest how they themselves have felt or behaved in similar circumstances. Peer group behaviors are strongly indicative of the patient's own current or future choices.

- Empathetic lead in
  A potentially anxiety-producing subject is introduced by a brief empathetic statement and then asks the patient to test the truth: "If I were in your situation... (problem briefly stated), I think I would feel this way... (description of what an expected reaction might be). Is this true for you?" When the provider is on target, the patient appreciates such perceptiveness and often acknowledges it with a smile, a nod, relaxation of tension, or direct verbal affirmation. The conversation easily flows from there. If the patient says, "It's not that way at all.", follow with "Tell me how it is for you, then?"

- Advance notice of understanding
  When delivered in an open and straightforward manner, comments such as "Many people your age smoke... Do you?" or "Many young people your age... (smoke pot, have sex, etc.). Where do you stand on this issue?" reassures the patient to not worry about a judgmental response.

Tips for Conducting a Successful Interview

Young Teens
- Use language they understand (concrete in nature) and expect concrete questions and answers.
- Help them in identifying their feelings.
- Realize that adolescents are very loyal to their friends and possibly in conflict with their parents.

Older Teens
- Can be treated like adults and the interview can be conducted without their parents or guardian present.
- Assess if the teen has moved from concrete to abstract thinking.
- Adolescents regress under stress. One day they appear to be very mature and responsible, the next, they could be immature and irresponsible.
- Allow the adolescent to identify his or her needs.

Overall
- Introduce yourself first: My name is ___; I am a Teen Health Provider.
- Address the teen by name.
- Respect their privacy and confidentiality (know the laws).
- Do not judge them.
- Ask questions that are open-ended.
- Assess developmental level.
- Listen for understanding, not truth.

Preventive Services Guidelines

Except for immunizations, few health professionals actually address prevention in a comprehensive manner with their adolescent and young adult patients. This is because professionals may have limited clinical time, inadequate reimbursement, or may lack specific training. They may also disagree as to the services and content that should be provided, or simply may not believe in the effectiveness of such prevention efforts. Lack of agreement between the adolescent and the clinician on the nature of the health concerns can also negatively affect outcomes. Youth barriers include the lack of available preventive services convenient to adolescents (such as schools and malls), the cost to an adolescent who may not be able to pay for services, and the adolescent's perception of lack of confidentiality in various settings. Although providing factual information to adolescents requires less time than interactive health guidance, and factual information is easier to give in a busy clinic, it is significantly less effective.

The health problems targeted by prevention recommendations represent an enormous cost to society. Providing preventive education will have a beneficial effect on youth health and should reduce the burden of suffering, but actual outcome effectiveness is not yet known. Conservative projections support the fact that even limited success in behavioral change and risk reduction will have profound and significant effects on populations of adolescents. Multiple opportunities and approaches need to be utilized and created to identify adolescents who have begun health risk behaviors or who have either physical or emotional disorders, and to provide and reinforce health promotion messages.

The American Medical Association's *Guidelines for Adolescent Preventive Services* (GAPS) recommends a complete physical examination only three times during adolescence, at ages 12, 16, and 19 or 20 years. However, GAPS recommends annual screening for health risk behaviors and providing health guidance.

Health Conditions Addressed by GAPS
    I. Promoting physical fitness
   II. Promoting healthy dietary habits and preventing eating disorders and obesity
  III. Promoting healthy psychosexual adjustment, and preventing the negative health
       consequences of sexual behaviors
   IV. Preventing the use of tobacco products
    V. Preventing the use and abuse of alcohol and other drugs
   VI. Preventing severe or recurrent depression and suicide
  VII. Preventing physical, sexual, and emotional abuse
 VIII. Preventing injury and promoting safety

Recommended Immunizations

TDAP boosters should be given at age 11 (if at least 5 years have passed since the last dose) and then a booster Td should be given every 10 years after the initial series is completed.

Hepatitis B series should be given to complete a three-dose regimen.

Measles, Mumps, and Rubella (MMR) should be given if there have not been two doses.

Human Papilloma Virus for females, in three doses which are 2 months and 4 months apart (recommendations for males may vary by country).

Varicella should be given to those without a history of clinical varicella disease or a positive titer.

Hepatitis A should be given in two doses that are 6 months apart.

Meningococcal vaccine (Menactra) may be given as early as age 11, but routinely at age 18 upon entry into college dormitories as well as other groups at increased risk such as military recruits.

Physical Health Screening

Routine physical examination should include an assessment of pubertal maturation and attention to the particular conditions listed below that are common during adolescence. Height, weight, and blood pressure should be measured. The body mass index is calculated to determine if the adolescent meets the criteria for a weight problem. Removing clothes in the office can be very stressful for adolescents, sometimes resulting in avoidance of health care. Most examinations will not require an adolescent to completely disrobe; in fact, nearly all of the examinations can be conducted with the patient clothed, and only removal of some clothes as required. Specific evaluation of the following areas on the physical examination should include:

- Skin
  Rashes, acne, piercings, tattoos. Complications of piercings and tattoos can include allergic dermatitis to metals or dyes, as well as keloids, and skin infections.
- Mouth/Teeth
  Caries, enamel erosion from tongue piercings. Tongue piercings can cause swelling, gingival injury, and tooth fractures as well as chipping.
- Musculoskeletal
  Osgood-Schlatters disease, scoliosis (especially in premenarchal females).
- Breast
  Gynecomastia in males. Sexual maturity rating in females, but teaching or doing a routine female breast examination is not necessary for early and middle adolescents with no concerns. Recent studies suggest that it is actually counterproductive to do routine breast examinations or teach breast self-examinations to adolescents.
- Genitourinary male
  Sexual maturity rating of pubic hair; assess for masses, hernia, varicocele, rash. (Those who are sexually experienced may have chlamydia screening performed by urine-DNA testing.)
- Genitourinary female
  Sexual maturity rating of pubic hair; assess for normal external anatomy and lesions. A pelvic examination is not necessary for a female who does not need a Pap test until age 21 and has no genitourinary symptoms. (Those who are sexually experienced should have STD testing performed by urine-DNA testing, and a vaginal swab without a speculum can be used for GC culture if no urine-DNA testing is available.) Without signs or symptoms, a speculum or bimanual examination is not necessary.

Laboratory Screening

Laboratory screening tests will vary by country and demographic needs and trends, but the following are considered minimum and routine:

- Anemia
  Hemoglobin screening for menstruating females during adolescence and in females with a history of iron deficiency anemia or polymenorrhagia.
- Lipids
  Adolescents up to age 18 should be screened for hyperlipidemia with a non-fasting total cholesterol when there is a parent with elevated cholesterol, or if there is a personal history of hypertension, obesity, or diabetes mellitus. Every young adult

aged 19 years and older should have one non-fasting total cholesterol. Screen an adolescent with a fasting lipid profile if a parent or grandparent was 55 years old or younger with documented myocardial infarction, angina, peripheral vascular disease, cerebrovascular disease, sudden cardiac death, or coronary atherosclerosis.

- Tuberculosis (TB) screening
  Questionnaires should be administered to determine the existence of risks below and if there is a history of receiving BCG or taking TB medications.
  Tuberculosis testing should be done when there is
  1. Contact with a person with known or suspected TB.
  2. Emigration or travel from or living in endemic countries.
  3. Significant contact with an individual from an endemic country.
  4. Radiologic or clinical evidence of TB.
     Note: For HIV-infected individuals, incarcerated youth, and user1s+– .- of illicit drugs, test annually.

- STD screening
  Screenings should be done for all sexually experienced females up to age 25 — test for chlamydia annually. Some recommendations also include males. Screen annually for gonorrhea in high-risk individuals, particularly those with more than one sexual partner. Chlamydia and gonorrhea screening is available by urine-based nucleic acid amplification testing, which permits noninvasive screening without a urethral swab or pelvic examination. A vaginal swab without a speculum can be used for GC culture if no urine-DNA testing is available. The experience of HIV screening and effective follow-up counseling should be offered to all sexually experienced adolescents, and may have profound behavioral effects.

- Papanicolaou (Pap) smear
  Pap smear should first be performed at age 21 regardless of sexual experience.

A 14-year-old female came to her doctor with her mother for treatment of a sore throat. The office routinely uses a risk screening questionnaire, and the clinician always meets with adolescents alone before parents join them for evaluation of acute illnesses. With the help of the questionnaire, a brief interview revealed sexual experience, both orally and vaginally. The clinician confidentially obtained and sent urine for both chlamydia and gonorrhea (GC)-DNA testing as well as an oral GC culture, and also recorded the patient's cell phone number. Her menses occurred 1 week prior to the visit, and she was not sexually active for over a month, but she did plan to be again soon, so she was given an injection of Depo-Provera. The mother was then invited into the examination room, and the chief complaint was reviewed, then the physical examination was done for a sore throat. A throat culture for strep was taken, and penicillin was prescribed. Two days later, the culture for strep was negative, the oral GC culture was positive, and the urine test for chlamydia test was positive. The patient was contacted confidentially, and the appropriate antibiotics were given, as well as a 6-week follow-up appointment for testing of cure for GC and chlamydia, as well as a pregnancy test before her next Depo-Provera injection.

Preventive Adolescent Risk Screening

Risk screening should be done at every health visit, including acute care visits. However, there must be a zone of safety in a health office. Many parents feel that they should be present during the interview, or at least need to be told information. It is important to make sure that parents fully understand why the safety zone in a health office is so important, and know that the health professional recognizes that parents are the most critical forces in adolescents' lives. Parents who are guided to understand the role of health personnel as an added safety net will welcome the opportunity. If the physician simply asks the parent to leave the room, the parent will feel as though they are being told "I can handle this better than you can." After the brief risk screening, the parent is then asked to join the physician and teen to discuss the chief complaint for an acute visit.

Patient and parent should fill out health screening questionnaires (see Table 1 and pages 248–249) on physical health and psychosocial issues prior to talking with the clinician. This can help focus the content of the encounter and facilitate the clinician's ability to address crucial issues when there are time constraints. The adolescent should complete the risk screening questionnaire in private to maintain confidentiality.

Table 1   Brief risk screening Teen Questionnaire

If you are 13 years old or more, when you come to the office we would like you to answer these questions yourself, privately. Please circle "Yes" or "No" and hand this to the doctor or health provider. It is private between you and the doctor.

1. In the last 6 months, have you driven or been in a car when the driver was drinking or on drugs? .... No Yes
2. Are you now taking any medicines, birth control pills, or other drugs?
   .... No Yes

3. Do you ever drink alcohol, smoke, or take other drugs (besides medications prescribed for you)? .... No Yes
4. Would you like birth control information or pamphlets? .... No Yes
5. Are you having problems at home, at school, or with friends? ..... No Yes
6. Do you currently have a male and/or female lover? (If "Yes," circle which one) .... No Yes
7. In the past 2 weeks have you felt down, depressed or hopeless? .... No Yes
8. Have you ever had genital sexual contact (including vaginal, anal or oral sex)? .... No Yes
9. Have you ever seriously thought about killing yourself, made a plan, or actually tried to kill yourself? .... No Yes
10. In the last month, did you ride in a vehicle without a seatbelt on? .... No Yes
11. Is there anything else you would like to discuss with the doctor or health provider? .... No Yes

[Adapted from Deisher R, Paperny D, 1982]

There are numerous versions of adolescent and parent surveys that clinicians can use in the office or clinic. Computerized assessments such as the Youth Health Program are discussed in Chapter 10. Office personnel must to be sensitive to the confidentiality needs of adolescents and enjoy working with this age group. Office fees pose a problem for providing confidential services when itemized insurance bills automatically are sent home to the parents. Adolescents may be able and willing to pay for confidential services. Sliding scale payment options have successfully facilitated access to care. Clinicians should also be aware of local free clinics and community services such as health departments or family planning clinics.

Risk Behaviors of Adolescents in Developed Countries

Violence, Injury and Abuse
- Violence and injury account for 3 out of 4 adolescent deaths.
- More than 3 out of 10 adolescents who die are killed in motor vehicle accidents. Half of these accidents involve alcohol.

Substance Use
- 70% have smoked cigarettes at least once.
- 90% of high school seniors have consumed alcohol at least once.
- 50% have tried marijuana; 15% have tried cocaine or methamphetamine.

Sexuality

- By the time they are 18 years old, 65% of boys and 50% of girls are sexually experienced.
- Half of American adolescents do not use contraceptives the first time they have intercourse.
- Half of all premarital pregnancies occur within the first 6 months of sexual initiation.
- 11% of adolescent girls become pregnant each year, and about 5% have abortions.

HIV/AIDS

- More than 2 out of 3 adolescents with AIDS were infected through sexual contact with adults.
- Although few patients with AIDS are between the ages of 13 and 19, the prevalence of HIV infection among young adults implies that infection during adolescence is common.

Mental Health and Disorders

- Millions of adolescents need mental health services but do not receive them.

General Physical Health

- Over 5% of adolescents are obese, and as much as a third are overweight.
- Perhaps 2% of adolescents have persistent hypertension, which is linked to heart disease and stroke as adults.

Below are the top risk issues of concern for which intervention has the most important effect and outcome for adolescents and alleviates the most personal and social costs as well as morbidity. They are in priority order but do not reflect severity. The severity is uncovered during interviews, which can determine the serious issues. You may find that other concerns (you initially thought were serious) may be less important. It is important that the provider not bias the screening process with their own personal priorities or for lack of time or comfort in dealing with sensitive issues.

Clinical Prioritization of Risk Behaviors (priority order, but not necessarily a severity order)

1. Affective issues, depression and suicide risk/lethality
2. Sexually experienced/active (abstinence; contraceptive needs; male condom non-use, desire for a baby; HIV risk; sex with alcohol/drugs)
3. Driving under the influence, riding with intoxicated drivers
4. Carrying weapons and guns
5. Substance abuse (other than alcohol and marijuana)

6. Sexual abuse, physical abuse
7. Abuse of alcohol
8. Seat belt non-use
9. Abuse of marijuana
10. Bicycle safety and helmet non-use
11. F: Pregnant and concurrent use of drugs and alcohol
12. M: Anabolic steroid use in bodybuilding
13. Sexual orientation, gender identity issues
14. Pregnant and inadequate prenatal care
15. Sexually transmitted diseases (other than HIV)
16. Gun safety at home
17. Anorexia and eating disorders
18. Violence exposure
19. Smoking: quitting tobacco
20. Inadequate exercise, fitness, overweight: weight management
21. Family issues
22. School performance, career choices
23. Communication skills and assertiveness, relationship problems
24. Stress management techniques

Synopsis of prioritization order for the top 10 identifiable problems
Suicide
Sex
Driving and riding under the influence
Carry guns
Hard drugs
Abuse
Alcohol
Seatbelts
Marijuana
Safety and helmets

You may wish to use an inverted HEADSSS examination list to remember most of the priority content of the psychosocial history:

S: Suicide — suicidal ideation, and other affective issues (including eating disorders)
S: Sexuality — dating, sexual activity, contraception, STDs, (sexual preference)
S: Safety — DUI/RUI, carrying guns (use of seatbelts, bike helmets)
D: Drugs — hard drug use and abuse

A: Abuse/Activities — recreation, peers and social activities (including alcohol and
     marijuana use)
E: Education — academic performance and vocational goals
H: Home — family relationships and living arrangements

Health Education

The aim of health education is not only to impart knowledge about healthy behavior and
to help motivate positive choices and changes, but also to develop the skills needed
to make changes. The timing and the content of such education must be based on
individual readiness. Optimal health education is both interactive and designed for
the developmental level and specific needs of each youth. Interactive multimedia can
accomplish some of these tasks, and adolescents are particularly responsive to this
format (see Chapter 9). Though counseling gives information on the long-term effects
of health risk behaviors, this is rarely motivational for youths. Use direct, current
information about a youth or his/her body — "Do you think cigarettes are yellowing
your teeth or making your clothes smell?" rather than "On cigarettes, you may die at
age 45 instead of 65."

The Health Provider's Role is to Optimize Health Outcomes, therefore

• Disapproval of behavior is unprofessional. Disagreement with poor choices is
  appropriate.
• Brief health advice "should's" and scare tactics rarely change behavior.
• Adolescents are in situations, making emotional choices which are not always under
  volitional control.
• The provider is obligated to refer adolescent patients that he or she is unable or
  unwilling to counsel.
• "Don't ask, don't tell" is inadequate health care.

    Because providing factual information to adolescents requires less time than an
interactive health guidance process, physicians often use this method of counseling
when faced with busy clinic schedules. The results of various studies, however, suggest
that providing information or advice alone is insufficient to promote behavioral changes
in adolescents [Prochaska *et al.*, 1992]. Health guidance is most effective when it is
interactive, that is, when the adolescent and physician have an opportunity to listen
to each other, express concerns about a particular issue, and jointly develop a plan of
action to address those concerns.
    Agreement by the physician and adolescent on the nature of health concerns can
have a positive effect on the clinical outcome. For example, a review of medical records

for 135 clinic visits found a total of 275 identified health problems [Starfield *et al.*, 1981]. The ways problems were communicated to the patients were categorized, and then the association to clinical outcomes was analyzed. Two-thirds of health problems identified by a physician alone showed little or no improvement at follow-up sessions. However, the same number of problems mutually agreed upon by both the physician and the patient showed improvement at follow-up sessions, regardless of the perceived severity or the type of problem. Brief Negotiation in brief clinical encounters is a collaborative, patient-centered method for increasing an adolescent's motivation to accomplish health behavior changes and to negotiate the best course of action (see Chapter 10).

Techniques for Improving the Effectiveness of Health Guidance

1. Define, with the adolescent, the nature and extent of the health-risk behaviors that are problematic.
2. Determine the adolescent's attitude towards the behavior, reasons for the behavior (if appropriate), his or her level of knowledge regarding possible consequences of the behavior, and motivation to change.
3. Reinforce healthy behaviors and health promotion messages from school, family, and the community.
4. Determine with the adolescent a concrete, personalized course of action.
5. Encourage the adolescent to commit to this plan, and provide positive reinforcement when success is achieved.

Anticipatory Guidance

Anticipatory guidance prepares youths for situations and challenges and helps them recognize potential problems later, as well as acquire information and attitudes needed for healthy lifestyles and for resisting health risk behaviors. Health guidance should encourage adolescents to maintain healthy lifestyles and to develop social skills they can use to resist peer pressure and make appropriate decisions about their health behaviors.

Many youths are skeptical and consider the advice of a provider subject to interpretation or bias, even if it is completely, factually correct and the conclusions are logical. The combined effect of computer-assisted instruction (see Chapter 9) with personal obstacle identification and problem solving can be an extraordinarily powerful intervention.

Guidance for parents of minors involve providing information about adolescent development and the signs of disease or emotional distress, exploring parenting behaviors, emphasizing the value of family activities, and reinforcing the importance of positive role models. Providers should identify parental concerns and questions, provide information, help parents determine better parenting strategies, and reinforce those that work. Family-centered intervention strategies are very useful.

Clinical Prioritization of Anticipatory Guidance
1. Relationships and sex
2. Avoiding drugs and substance abuse
3. Avoiding alcohol and tobacco
4. Personal safety and injury reduction
5. Eating right, exercise and fitness
6. The Six Achievable Adolescent Behavior Goals (see page 250)

Three Adolescent Care Principles
1. Adolescents do want to discuss most health topics with their health care providers but may be unable to begin the discussion.
2. Parents do want health care providers to discuss most health topics with their adolescents.
3. Ensuring confidentiality is important in facilitating open communication with adolescents, particularly about sensitive topics such as sexuality and substance use.

Confidentiality

A general rule in adolescent health is that confidentiality in communications is the *sine qua non* between provider and patient. Nearly every jurisdiction will have one or more laws permitting minors to consent to health care based on the conditions involved (STDs, pregnancy, contraception, substance abuse). Many have laws enabling minors to consent to all health care if they are emancipated or mature minors. Emancipation includes minors living away from home and managing their own financial affairs, minors in the armed services, minors who are or have been pregnant and minors who are parents. Mature minors demonstrate the cognitive maturity to be able to voluntarily decide on consent to treatment.

There are certainly exceptions to maintaining confidentiality. These primarily relate to matters where the adolescent could seriously harm or kill themselves (suicide) or others, or where state laws require the reporting of abuse (sexual or physical); child abuse laws include all minors. In cases of abuse, however, most adolescents readily agree to parental disclosure and indeed want protection. From a management point of view, parents must often be involved with pregnant teens who intend to give birth, and with those who have significant substance abuse problems. Here, too, it usually is not difficult to obtain the minor's consent after the reality has been introduced.

A major obstacle to providing adolescent health care has often been the lack of clearly defined local statutes on confidentiality, consent, and other subtle legal issues. Even different practice settings within the same community often have different approaches to the issue of confidentiality. Because local laws often differ, this discussion will only feature general principles. Specific situations regarding patients may require the advice of an attorney.

One school of thought suggests adolescents need to be told explicitly before an interview that confidentiality will be abrogated if there is a life-threatening situation, if there is a reporting law, if health is otherwise likely to be compromised, or if the problem cannot be adequately handled alone or in collaboration with the health provider. Another approach is to speak from a sincere and concerned point of view and imply confidentiality with good judgment, unless specifically asked by a youth, since itemization of breach situations in advance may close off the most important communication. Simply put, "Unless it's not safe or it's an emergency, I will keep your information private."

To interact effectively with a minor, the provider must have some level of understanding about patient confidentiality. As a youth matures, the provider should increase the level of confidentiality as there is increased ability to thoughtfully engage and give informed consent to evaluation and intervention plans. This may change the provider's relationship with the parent, particularly if there is a long-standing relationship with the family. A provider should explain the need for increased privacy and confidentiality to parents in advance, and explain limits of privacy when appropriate. The developmental stage as well as the onset and progress of the tasks of adolescence must always supercede the chronological age in determining the level of parental involvement in an adolescent's health care.

Stages of Adolescent Health Care

1. Pre-adolescence = parent primary, child secondary
2. Early adolescence = parent-adolescent collaboration
3. Mid-adolescence = adolescent primary, parent secondary
4. Late adolescence = adolescent primary, parent optional

The *parent-adolescent collaboration* approach is appropriate for early adolescents, prior to the emergence of emancipation issues, where the parent and adolescent are addressed together for obtaining the history and developing a treatment plan. Both are present in the examination room at the same time and share in the decision-making process.

The *adolescent primary/parent secondary* approach is for middle adolescents at the beginning of emancipation. The adolescent is primarily addressed by the clinician, has private time with the clinician to discuss confidential issues, and has the initial discussions about the treatment plan with the clinician. The parent then joins them to review the visit. It is often useful for the adolescent to describe the non-confidential details and plans to the parent as this contributes to self-esteem and self-sufficiency. It is particularly important to allow adolescents with chronic illnesses to have a role in their treatment decisions.

The *adolescent primary/parent optional* approach is for late adolescents who are ready to assume responsibility for their own health care. In this case, the clinician does not communicate directly with the parent unless there is concern about harm (e.g. suicide). It is the responsibility of the patient to relay information to the parent.

The Physician's Role in Maintaining and Breaching Confidentiality

Confidentiality is crucial in providing proper health care to adolescents. Frank discussions between health care providers and adolescents are most likely to occur when the adolescents have private time alone without parents. Teens that have private time with providers are much more likely to reveal risk behaviors and ask questions. The need for privacy is usually related to the specific medical issue. Adolescents are rarely concerned about parental knowledge about a routine physical, an acute febrile illness, or a weight problem. However, adolescents are much less likely to want to disclose information and are more likely to express concern about parental knowledge regarding sensitive topics such as sexuality, substance use, and mental health. If parental notification were required, only 45% of American adolescents report they would seek services for depression, 19% for birth control, 15% for STI treatment, and 17% for treatment of drug use. When assured of confidentiality, the figure rose: 57% would seek care for depression, 64% for contraceptive services, 65% for STIs, and 66% for drug use. At Planned Parenthood in Wisconsin, USA, 60% of teens would stop using reproductive health services, including STD testing, if their parents had to be notified by legal mandate. Educating adolescents about the health care services they can receive without their parents' knowledge increases the probability that teens will seek and receive preventive counseling and screening.

No single legal issue affects teenagers and clinicians more than the issue of confidentiality. It is in the minds of adolescent patients — even if they are being seen for a trivial illness as they place a very high value on confidentiality. Six out of 10 adolescents have health concerns that they would want to keep private from their parents, and 1 in 4 would avoid health care for those concerns if it meant that their parents might find out. Nearly half would not go to their regular physician for pregnancy, STD, or substance abuse concerns [Cheng *et al.*, 1993]. Numerous laws, public health regulations, and court decisions now recognize an adolescent's right to confidential health care. Licensed health care professionals can often counsel and treat adolescents without parental knowledge or consent under statutory and common law. They are legally allowed "privileged communication" by the rules of professional privilege which may not apply to non-professionals. However, liability for health outcomes is often a factor in practice styles, though there are no known documented cases of liability being assessed where a clinician has provided quality services in good faith. Nearly every jurisdiction has consent laws that address the confidentiality of minors. United States courts have struck down laws that mandated parental consent for minors to obtain contraceptives.

The problem of access to care for sensitive issues is made worse by clinicians who inappropriately guarantee unconditional confidentiality. Confusion can also occur when the front desk office staff do not deliver the same confidentiality messages as the clinicians. Written policies on adolescent confidentiality improve consistency within an office or clinic. Providing confidential services including reproductive health and substance abuse counseling can increase patient satisfaction and expand the capability of a primary care office. However, it is important to recognize that some adolescents may choose to seek confidential services elsewhere because they feel safer in an environment where they can be more anonymous.

The easiest way to establish these principles in a clinical practice is to anticipate. When a child reaches age 12, a handout can be provided to parents explaining that with the 13th birthday, certain confidential health care can be provided. When discussed in advance, the idea of confidentiality does not bother many parents, but if it has to be raised in an emergency (e.g. parents find a teenager's birth control pills), then problems may occur. In practice, the term "confidentiality" may actually not be used. Instead, clinicians can explain to teenagers using the word "private" or a statement such as "Whatever you tell me will stay between us, unless there could be harm to yourself or someone else."

There are also specific laws about mandatory reporting of sexual or physical abuse and certain infectious diseases including STDs. When the clinician feels that a particular issue falls into the disclosure category, it is important that the adolescent is told about the need for disclosure before informing the parent.

If the clinician believes that the circumstance is an emergency or dangerous, he or she may disclose confidential information to parents after consulting with the adolescent or making a good faith effort to do so. Clinicians may release such information at their discretion when extenuating circumstances warrant disclosure of selected confidential information, for example, when it is perceived to be in the best interest of the adolescent to do so (i.e. child is missing).

Confidentiality is not absolute. Nor does it mean that clinicians should not encourage their patients to discuss sensitive medical problems with their parents when it is appropriate and safe to do so. There are instances in which confidentiality must be breached:

- If a teenager is in imminent danger of harming him- or herself or someone else. This is when a clinician may need to call the police rather than an agency.
- If a teenager has been sexually or physically abused.
- If a teenager has a reportable STD. Teens need to be informed that they are being reported to the public health department.
- If there is a specific local statute that mandates disclosure.

If the particular jurisdiction permits adolescents to consent to health care on their own or the parent has assented to confidential services, then the parent does not have a right to the health information in the medical record regarding that particular medical problem. Whether parents can access this information depends upon local or other applicable law. Physicians caring for adolescents constantly juggle the best interests of adolescents and their families. Open, honest communication between adolescents and their families is usually the best way to resolve conflict on these difficult issues. Parents can be invited to a three-way conversation with the clinician and adolescent with the understanding that certain information cannot be revealed without the consent of the adolescent unless the potential for significant harm has been determined. Seeing teenage patients should not involve major legal risks if clinicians follow standard procedures for confidential care.

Standard Procedures for Adolescent Health Care
- Know local applicable law.
- Consult with local and hospital attorneys when questions arise.
- Carefully document information thoroughly in the medical record (with the exception of sensitive or confidential material that should be carefully marked).
- With informed consent by the mature minor, document cognitive levels, mental status and ability to understand and weigh the risks of treatment.
- Obtain a second opinion if needed.
- Always do what is best for the patient. This approach is least likely to result in legal difficulties since courts usually view this as the physician's appropriate role in treating patients.

Consent and Treatment

At certain ages, in certain jurisdictions, and for certain types of care, consent by the adolescent is required for the release of information pertaining to:

1. Family planning services (i.e. pregnancy, birth control)
2. STD
3. HIV/AIDS
4. Alcohol/substance abuse and treatment

The adolescent's expressed written consent is required to release them to any party (including parents).

Although adolescents under legal age are minors, there are precedents which permit them to consent to health services:

- Emergency care
  Emergency care can be provided to teenagers (and even younger children) without parental consent. Parents should be contacted as soon as possible in such situations. How an emergency is defined may vary by jurisdiction, but in general, courts have given a wide latitude to health professionals, especially if efforts to contact parents have been documented. Emergencies may not necessarily be life-threatening — a teen with a broken leg or bleeding would almost certainly qualify. In general, when clinicians act in the patient's best interests, the law is not a problem.
- Emancipated minors
  They are usually (depending on the jurisdiction) those serving in the armed forces or living away from home apart from their parents, and managing their own financial affairs or self-supporting. They also include teens who are married, pregnant or are already parents, including minors who are divorced.
- Living on their own and not self-supporting
  Even if they are not self-supporting, minors can often consent for their own treatment if they are living apart from their parents with parental consent.
- Mature minors
  They are those who demonstrate sufficient cognitive maturity to understand the risks and benefits of proposed medical treatments and alternatives, and can voluntarily decide on consent. The mature minor doctrine is from common law (case law). It means that a physician can provide medical care to a minor when that care is routine, not high-risk, non-negligent, and the minor is capable of providing informed consent. Often, this is a teenager who is near the age of consent. A few jurisdictions have actually enacted specific legislation to accept this doctrine. This is not helpful with

the issue of treating immature minors who may want or need confidential health care.

- Incarcerated youth
  Some jurisdictions specifically allow incarcerated youth to consent for their own health care.
- Medical condition emancipation
  Statutes will specify when minors may consent for pregnancy care, contraception, STD treatment, alcohol and drug abuse treatment, as well as some mental health counseling and treatment as follows:

  — Most jurisdictions allow minors to consent for evaluation and treatment of sexually transmitted diseases. This is because public health outweighs the parents' right to know about their teens.
  — Most jurisdictions also have specific statutes allowing minors to consent for contraceptive services. Some statutes qualify that the minor would suffer harm without the services being provided. If no local law exists, a minor may still be able to consent, based on the mature minor doctrine and a constitutional right to privacy. Many courts have struck down statutes that attempted to require parental consent for the provision of contraception.

- Most jurisdictions have legislation that allows minors who are pregnant to consent for their pregnancy-related care.
- Many jurisdictions have passed laws enabling minors to consent for treatment for the abuse of alcohol or other drugs.
- Many jurisdictions have legislation mandating either parental notification or parental consent before an adolescent can undergo an abortion, and some include a judicial bypass route where a judge can rule that a minor is mature and able to make her own abortion decision. Statutes sometimes include exceptions for emergencies, incest, or abuse.

Legal Pointers in Adolescent Health
1. Do what is best for the patient — there is never a guarantee against legal actions, but you will be at an advantage.
2. In an emergency, care for the patient first, and worry about the legalities later.
3. Providing contraception to a minor is probably universally legal and defensible — physicians are not successfully sued for prescribing birth control to minors.

Every contact with an adolescent, including an acute care visit, is an opportunity for risk screening, intervention, and promotion of their well-being and better health choices. Although adolescents who come for acute health care do not necessarily expect to be asked about their behaviors, it can become an expected routine. As you read the following chapters, consider that your role is to continually optimize adolescents' personal choices and behaviors, and you are thereby addressing the issues that put adolescents at the greatest health risks.

Suggested Readings and Bibliography

Ackard DM, Neumark-Sztainer D. (2001). Health care information sources for adolescents: age and gender differences on use, concerns and needs. *J Adolesc Health*, 29, pp. 170–176.

American Medical Association, Council on Scientific Affairs. (1993). Confidential health services for adolescents. *JAMA*, 269, pp. 1420–1424.

American School Health Association. (1989). *National Adolescent Student Health Survey.*

Cheng TL, Savageau JA, Sattler AL, *et al.* (1993). Confidentiality in health care: a survey of knowledge, perceptions and attitudes among high school students. *JAMA*, 269, pp. 1404–1407.

Cohen MI. (1994). Adolescents: left behind by our health-care system. *Contemporary Adol Gyn* (Summer ed.), pp. 6–11.

Crockenberg S, Soby B. (1989). Self-esteem and teenage pregnancy. In: Mecca AM, Smelser NJ, Vasconcellos J (eds), *The Social Importance of Self-esteem*, pp. 125–164. (University of California Press, Berkeley).

Deisher R, Paperny D. (1982). Variations in sexual behavior of adolescents. In: Kelley VC (ed), *Brenemann – Practice of Pediatrics*, Chapter 25. (Harper & Row, Philadelphia).

Downs SM, Klein JD. (1995). Clinical preventive services efficacy and adolescents' risky behaviors. *Arch Pediat Adolesc Med*, 149, pp. 374–379.

Dryfoos JG. (1998). *Safe Passage: Making It Through Adolescence in a Risky Society.* (Oxford University Press, New York).

Elster AB. (1993). Confronting the crisis in adolescent health: visions for change. *J Adolesc Health*, 14, pp. 505–508.

Elster AB, Kuznets NJ. (1994). *AMA Guidelines for Adolescent Preventive Services (GAPS): Recommendations and Rationale.* (Williams & Wilkins, Baltimore).

Fisher M. (1992). Parents' views of adolescent health issues. *Pediatrics*, 90, pp. 335–341.

Fleming M (ed). (1996). *Healthy Youth 2000: A Mid-Decade Review.* (American Medical Association, Department of Adolescent Health, Chicago).

Gans JE (ed). (1993). *Policy Compendium on Confidential Health Services for Adolescents.* (American Medical Association, Chicago).

Gans JE, Alexander B, Chu RC, *et al.* (1995). The cost of comprehensive preventive medical services for adolescents. *Arch Pediatr Adolesc Med*, 149, pp. 1226–1234.

Ginsburg KR, Menapace AS, Slap GB. (1997). Factors affecting the decision to seek primary care: the voice of adolescents. *Pediatrics*, 100, pp. 922–930.

Ginsburg KR, Slap GB, Cnaan A, *et al.* (1995). Adolescents' perceptions of factors affecting their decisions to seek health care. *JAMA*, 273, pp. 1913–1918.

Green ME. (1994). *Bright Futures, Guidelines for Health Supervision of Infants, Children, and Adolescents.* (National Center for Education in Maternal and Child Health, Arlington).

Haggerty RJ. (1975). The new morbidity. In: Haggerty RJ, Roghmann KJ, Pless IB (eds), *Child Health and the Community*. (John Wiley & Sons, New York).

Halpern-Felsher BL, Ozer EM, Millstein SG, *et al.* (2000). Preventive services in a health maintenance organization: how well do pediatricians screen and educate adolescent patients?
Arch Pediatr Adolesc Med, 154, pp. 173–179.

Hawaii Department of Health. (1991). Adolescent Health in Hawaii: The Adolescent Health
Network's Teen Health Advisor Report. (Hawaii Department of Health, Honolulu).

Hoffman AD. (1980). A rational policy toward consent and confidentiality in adolescent care.
J Adolesc Health Care, 1, pp. 9–17.

Hofmann AD, Greydanus DE (eds). (1997). In: *Adolescent Medicine*. 3rd Edn. (McGraw-
Hill/Appleton & Lange, USA). ISBN-10: 0838500676; ISBN-13: 978-0838500675.

Klein JD, Allan MJ, Elster AB, *et al.* (2001). Improving adolescent preventive care in community
health centers. *Pediatrics*, 107, pp. 318–327.

McAuliffe TL, Difranceisco W, Reed BR. (2007). Effects of question format and collection
mode on the accuracy of retrospective surveys of health risk behavior: a comparison with
daily sexual activity diaries. *Health Psychol*, 26, pp. 60–67.

Neinstein LS. (2002). *Adolescent Health Care*. (Lippincott, Williams and Willkins,
Philadelphia).

Nelson CS, Wissow LS, Cheng TL. (2003). Effectiveness of anticipatory guidance: recent devel-
opments. *Curr Opin Pediatr*, 15, pp. 630–635.

Paperny DM. (1988). Teen Health Computer Programs, presented at AMA First National
Congress on Adolescent Health: *Charting a Course Through Turbulent Times*. Chicago,
USA.

Paperny DM. (1989). Children respond to computer-delivered health education. *American
Academy of Pediatrics News*, 5, p. 14.

Paperny DM. (1991). HMO innovations Video-enhanced medical advice. *HMO Practice*, 5,
pp. 212–213.

Paperny DM. (1992). Pediatric medical advice enhanced with use of video. *Am J Dis Child*,
146, pp. 785–786.

Paperny DM. (1994). Automated adolescent preventative services using computer-assisted video
multimedia. *J Adolesc Health*, 15, p. 66.

Paperny DM, Aono JY, Lehman RM, *et al.* (1988). Computer-assisted detection, evaluation, and
referral of sexually abused adolescents. *J Adolesc Health Care*, 9, p. 260.

Paperny DM, Starn JR. (1989). Adolescent pregnancy prevention by health education computer
games: computer-assisted instruction of knowledge and attitudes. *Pediatrics*, 83, pp. 742–
752.

Perrone J. (1988). Breaking barriers: computerized teen questionnaire eases discomfort with
sex issues. *American Medical News*, pp. 15–16.

Ponton LE. (1998). *The Romance of Risk: Why Teenagers Do the Things They Do.* (Basic Books,
USA).

Prochaska JO, DiClemente CC, Norcross JC. (1992). In search of how people change: applications to addictive behaviors. *Amer Psychologist*, 47, pp. 1102–1114.

Prochaska JO, Velicer WF, Rossi JS, *et al.* (1994). Stages of change and decisional balance for
12 problem behaviors. *Health Psychol*, 13, pp. 39–46.

Resnick M, Blum RW, Hedin D. (1980). The appropriateness of health services for adolescents:
youths' opinions and attitudes. *J Adolesc Heath Care*, 1, pp. 137–141.

Rosen D, Elster A, Hedberg V, *et al.* (1997). Clinical preventive services for adolescents: position
paper of the society for adolescent medicine. *J Adolesc Health*, 21, pp. 203–214.

Sobal J, Klein H, Graham D, *et al.* (1988). Health concerns of high school students and teachers' beliefs about student health concerns. *Pediatrics*, 81, pp. 218–223.

Society for Adolescent Medicine. (2004). Confidential health care for adolescents: position paper of the society for adolescent medicine. *J Adolesc Heath*, 35, pp. 160–167.

Starfield B, Wray C, Hess K, *et al.* (1981). The influence of patient-practitioner agreement on outcome of care. *Am J Public Health*, 71, pp. 127–131.

US Public Health Service. (1994). *The Clinician's Handbook of Preventive Services: Put Prevention into Practice.* (International Medical Publishing, Inc., Alexandria).

US Preventive Services Task Force. (1996). *Guide to Clinical Preventive Services: Report of the US Preventive Services Task Force.* 2nd edn. (Williams & Wilkins, Baltimore).

Walker Z, Townsend J, Oakley L, *et al.* (2002). Health promotion for adolescents in primary care: randomized controlled trial. *BMJ*, 325, p. 524.

Suggested Websites

The International Association for Adolescent Health (IAAH) is a multidisciplinary, non-government organization with a broad focus on youth health. This site describes IAAH principles, organization, conference schedules, activities and the current newsletter: http://www.iaah.org/index.html.

This site includes details about the American Medical Association (AMA) Guidelines for Adolescent Preventive Services (GAPS), a publications list — journal articles, news releases — and an extensive list of links for professionals, parents and teens: http://www.ama-assn.org/ama/pub/physician-resources/public-health/promoting-healthy-lifestyles/adolescent-health.shtml.

Chapter 2

Growth and Development

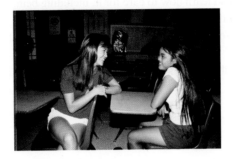

There is nothing but Consciousness: $C = E = mc^2$

Overview

Adolescence is not only filled with changes, it is filled with challenges as well. It is a period of rapid development with changes in body shape and size. In addition to the physical changes that occur, there is progress in maturation of cognitive, psychological, and social abilities. Puberty is the time between childhood and adulthood. Adolescence is a *biopsychosocial* process with *cognitive changes* that start before the beginning of secondary sexual characteristics, and they continue beyond the period of sexual maturity and the end of physical growth. For an adolescent to enter adulthood successfully, there are five (basic) tasks they will need to accomplish. They do not accomplish all these things in one stage, but most teens reach most of these goals by the time they are in late adolescence, yet some are delayed into young adulthood.

Joi is a 13-year-old female who presents for a routine examination for sports. Her past medical history and family history are unremarkable. She asks when she is "going to grow" and also wants to know why her periods have not yet started, stating that all of her friends are taller than she is and are having their periods. On physical examination, you note that she has Tanner 3 breasts and pubic hair.

Five Tasks of Adolescence
1. Develop abstract thinking skills, changing from concrete to abstract thought in cognitive development.
2. Achieve independence from family by becoming emotionally and physically independent.
3. Accept the body and learn how to care for it, including being responsible for one's own personal health care.
4. Begin to prepare for work after completion of school, and choosing a vocation or career.
5. Become comfortable with sexuality, and achieving maturity about their own sexuality.

Core functional areas for adolescent development
- Cognitive
- Social/emotional
- Physical
- Cultural
- Civic
- Vocational
- Moral/spiritual

Expected outcomes of adolescent development
- Competence
- Character
- Connection
- Confidence
- Contribution

Physical Growth

The hormonal onset of puberty depends on the production and interaction of various hormones, beginning in the hypothalamus. Increased gonadotropin-releasing hormone

(GNRH) releases follicle-stimulating hormone (FSH) and luteinizing hormone (LH). These cause the production of sex steroids (estrogen and testosterone), which facilitate secondary sex characteristics and changes in the body.

Feedback of estrogen in females causes more release of GNRH, allowing LH to begin ovulation. LH in males causes release of testosterone, leading to the development of secondary sexual characteristics. In both genders, secretion of sex steroids from the adrenal gland increases dehydroepiandosterone (DHEA), and this leads to development of pubic hair, body odor, and changes in the sebaceous glands. Activation of growth hormone (GH) causes an increase in growth velocity; together with increased insulin secretion, this increases somatic growth. Other hormones required for normal growth in adolescence are thyroid hormones and cortisol. Physical growth of puberty is a delicate interaction between the endocrine and skeletal systems. Increased secretion of GH, adrenal androgens, thyroid hormones, or estrogen can cause advanced bone maturation, and a deficiency of these hormones may delay it. The age of puberty may continue to decrease with the increased prevalence of obesity, as will be discussed in Chapter 4.

Puberty begins 2 years later in males than in females. The growth spurt can last 2 to 3 years, but occurs earlier in females, and their peak height velocity (PHV) is less, so their adult height is usually shorter than males. Both growth hormone and sex steroids add to the increase in linear velocity during which girls gain an average of 25 cm and boys gain an average of 28 cm. Epiphyseal closure marks the end of the growth spurt, and is 2 years later in males. During puberty, adipose tissue increases in females, so lean body mass decreases, but in males it increases from androgen effects.

There are dramatic physical changes in early adolescents. They are very interested in their pubertal changes. These dramatic biological changes may create feelings of insecurity and vulnerability, and raise teens' *sensitivity* to many concerns. There is uncertainty about appearance, and comparisons are often made of one's body to peers. Body image issues may develop. Interest in sexual anatomy and physiology is common, and worries occur about menstruation or nocturnal emissions, masturbation, and breast or penis size. During *middle adolescence*, boys have their growth spurt, an increase in muscle mass, and complete sexual development. Most girls' physical growth is complete 2 years after menarche. By *late adolescence*, adult physical growth is reached.

Sexual Development

The sexual maturity ratings (SMR) described by Marshall and Tanner [Tanner, 1962] are based on pubic hair and genital development in males, and pubic hair and breast development in females. It is not uncommon to have variation between the stage of breast/genital and pubic hair development in the same individual since they are controlled by different hormonal systems. Individual variation in the time of the beginning of puberty and the time between the different stages is dependent on nutrition and inheritance, but the progress of development is usually consistent within most races. The usual age of onset of puberty in North America is 9 to 14 years in boys and has not changed much in the last few decades. But the age of onset of puberty in females varies, with some African girls beginning puberty at 6 years old and Caucasian girls with signs at 7 years of age. Therefore, a female of those races who is otherwise healthy, with no evidence of neurological or chronic disease, who begins breast or pubic hair development at those ages, can be observed and not extensively evaluated. Asian females tend to be later in onset.

Male puberty begins with testicular enlargement, then adrenarche, penile enlargement, and peak height velocity (PHV). Spermarche usually occurs about 1 year after the beginning of puberty, with ejaculation at SMR level 3. The time for completion of male puberty averages 3 years, usually taking 2 to 5 years, and sexual maturity is usually reached by 17 years of age.

Telarche (breast buds) is normally the first sign of female puberty, but some girls begin with adrenarche. Telarche can start as late as age 14. Adrenarche then produces pubic and axillary hair, which is followed by PHV, then menarche. Menarche occurs about a year after PHV and by pubic hair stage 4 in half of girls. Ovulatory cycles might not occur until 3 years later, but fertility is present within 2 years of menarche, usually by age 15 years in most countries.

The objective description of physical pubertal development by Tanner is the widely accepted way to observe clinical progress. See Figures 2.1–2.3.

Breast development
- B1: Prepubertal — elevation of the papilla only.
- B2: Breast buds are noted or palpable with enlargement of the areola.
- B3: Further enlargement of the breast and areola with no separation of their contours.
- B4: Projection of areola and papilla to form a secondary mound over the rest of the breast.
- B5: Mature breast with projection of papilla only.

Female pubic hair development
- PH1: Prepubertal — no pubic hair.
- PH2: Sparse growth of long, straight or slightly curly, minimally pigmented hair, mainly on the labia.
- PH3: Considerably darker and coarser hair spreading over the mons pubis.

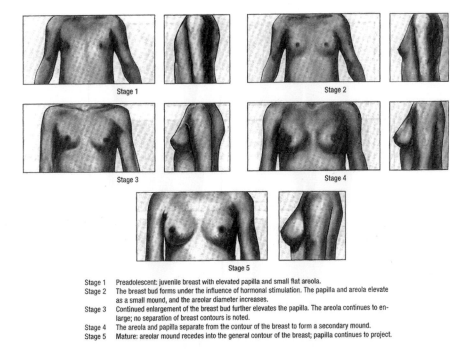

Stage 1   Preadolescent: juvenile breast with elevated papilla and small flat areola.
Stage 2   The breast bud forms under the influence of hormonal stimulation. The papilla and areola elevate as a small mound, and the areolar diameter increases.
Stage 3   Continued enlargement of the breast bud further elevates the papilla. The areola continues to enlarge; no separation of breast contours is noted.
Stage 4   The areola and papilla separate from the contour of the breast to form a secondary mound.
Stage 5   Mature: areolar mound recedes into the general contour of the breast; papilla continues to project.

Fig. 2.1   Tanner staging in females, breast development (Kamboj, 2010).

- PH4: Thick adult-type hair that does not yet spread to the medial surface of the thighs.
- PH5: Hair is adult in type and is distributed in the classic inverse triangle.

Male genital development
- G1: Preadolescent.
- G2: The testes are more than 2.5 cm in the longest diameter, and the scrotum is thinning and reddening.
- G3: Growth of the penis occurs in width and length, and further growth of the testes is noted.
- G4: Penis is further enlarged and testes are larger with a darker scrotal skin color.
- G5: Genitalia are adult in size and shape.

Male pubic hair development
- P1: Preadolescent — no pubic hair.

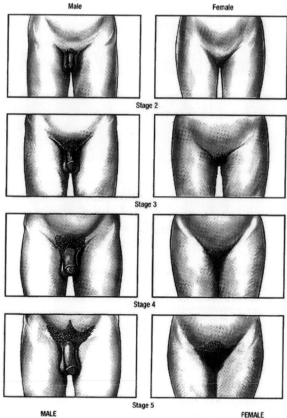

Fig. 2.2 Tanner staging in males and females, pubic hair development (Kamboj, 2010).

	MALE	FEMALE
Stage 1	Preadolescent: no pubic hair present; a fine vellus hair covers the genital area.	Preadolescent: no pubic hair present; a fine vellus hair covers the genital area.
Stage 2	A sparse distribution of long, slightly pigmented hair appears at the base of the penis.	A sparse distribution of long, slightly pigmented straight hair appears bilaterally along medial border of the labia majora.
Stage 3	The pubic hair pigmentation increases; the hairs begin to curl and to spread laterally in a scanty distribution.	The pubic hair pigmentation increases; the hairs begin to curl and to spread sparsely over the mons pubis.
Stage 4	The pubic hairs continue to curl and become coarse in texture. An adult type of distribution is attained, but the number of hairs remains fewer.	The pubic hairs continue to curl and become coarse in texture. The number of hairs continues to increase.
Stage 5	Mature: the pubic hair attains an adult distribution with spread to the surface of the medial thigh. Pubic hair will grow along linea alba in 80% of males.	Mature: pubic hair attains an adult feminine triangular pattern, with spread to the surface of the medial thigh.

- P2: Sparse growth of slightly pigmented, slightly curved pubic hair mainly at the base of the penis.
- P3: Thicker, curlier hair spread to the mons pubis.
- P4: Adult-type hair that does not yet spread to the medial thighs.
- P5: Adult-type hair spread to the medial thighs.

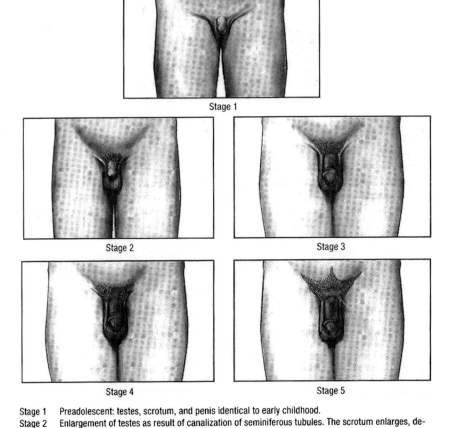

Stage 1

Stage 2 Stage 3

Stage 4 Stage 5

Stage 1 Preadolescent: testes, scrotum, and penis identical to early childhood.
Stage 2 Enlargement of testes as result of canalization of seminiferous tubules. The scrotum enlarges, developing a reddish hue and altering its skin texture. The penis enlarges slightly.
Stage 3 The testes and scrotum continue to grow. The length of the penis increases.
Stage 4 The testes and scrotum continue to grow; the scrotal skin darkens. The penis grows in width, and the glans penis develops.
Stage 5 Mature: adult size and shape of testes, scrotum, and penis.

Fig. 2.3 Tanner staging in males, genital development (Kamboj, 2010).

Delayed Puberty

Puberty is delayed if sexual maturation is prepubertal stage 1 at age 14 for males or in females at age 13. About 3% of healthy teens (primarily boys) will have pubertal delay, and most will have no pathology identified. Constitutional delay of puberty is due to delayed GNRH secretion, and family history often identifies a parent or sibling with delayed onset of puberty. Laboratory tests are normal and a bone age radiograph will be chronologically delayed but consistent with the stage of pubertal maturation. Final adult height will often be normal or high.

The history should screen for thyroid disorders, chronic illness, and family members with delayed puberty. The physical examination evaluates early (unnoticed) signs of sexual development (any breast buds in females, testicular volume > 4 ml in males) and any signs of chronic illness or congenital syndromes. Laboratory tests may include basic screening of CBC, ESR, TSH, and prolactin levels, but a karyotype should also be obtained if any signs of Klinefelter's or Turner's syndrome are noted. More extensive workup may include a bone age radiograph and serum gonadotropins to evaluate gonadal failure, where LH/FSH are high, compared to GNRH deficiency or constitutional delay, where LH/FSH are normal or low. A brain MRI may be ordered when clinically indicated.

Reassurances, anticipatory guidance and follow-up are the best approach for constitutional delay, particularly if there are signs of pubertal development. In the presence of psychosocial stressors, chronic illnesses, or disordered eating or exercising, use a multidisciplinary approach addressing health and nutrition. Endocrine disorders and proposed hormone treatments should be managed by an endocrine specialist. Complete discussion and evaluation of precocious and delayed puberty, growth disorders and other endocrine and chromosomal conditions can be found in most standard textbooks.

> Later in the course of your history, you find out that Joi has tried tobacco, drinks alcohol "on weekends with friends" and "smokes weed once in a blue moon." She denies a history of any sexual intercourse.

Psychosocial Development and Behavior

Every adolescent worldwide experiences a personal variation of typical psychosocial development, which is affected by culture, family, society and pubertal development. It can be stressful, but most adolescents do well during this non-uniform developmental process. The clinician who understands a patient's psychosocial developmental level can facilitate health-promoting choices and prevent much adolescent morbidity. Optimal communication with teens requires a complete understanding of psychosocial development in order to use questions, explanations, and health education adjusted to developmental level.

There are three types of *psychological autonomy* that adolescents strive for:

- *Emotional autonomy* is the establishment of close relationships. Adolescents begin to give consideration to the needs and wants of others, and weigh personal priorities (e.g. "Do I go out with my boy/girlfriend and skip going to the movie with my friends?").
- *Behavioral autonomy* is the ability to make independent decisions and follow through on them. Adolescents usually turn to peers for advice about friends and social matters, teachers and other adults for objective information, and parents for values and future plans (e.g. "Do I smoke cigarettes and drink beer to fit in with my friends?").
- *Value autonomy* is the development of a set of principles about right and wrong. They may challenge family and societal values (e.g. "My mom tells me not to drink, but sometimes she drinks at parties and drives home. Why is it okay for her to do it?").

As thinking abilities move from concrete to abstract thought, the adolescent can translate experiences into abstract ideas and think about the consequences of actions. Due to the common issue of adolescent *egocentrism*, there are four processes that maturing adolescents may resort to:

- Imaginary audience
  Abstract thinking allows a teen to consider what others are thinking. At the same time, the adolescent is concerned about bodily changes occurring at puberty. These physical changes, coupled with new thinking abilities, create for them the idea that everyone is thinking about them and looking at them.
- Personal fable
  "If everyone is watching you and thinking about you (the imaginary audience), then you must be someone special." This fable is the concept that one's thoughts and feelings are unique, and that some of the laws of nature do not apply to oneself (e.g. He will never grow old; she won't get pregnant or get an STD if she has unprotected intercourse).
- Hypocrisy
  This is the notion that rules apply differently to the adolescent than they do to others: An adolescent may feel that he should have free access to his parent's car, stereo or computer, while stating that when his parents come into his room, it is an invasion of his privacy.
- Overthinking
  This involves making things more complicated than they really are. An adolescent may attribute complicated motives to simple oversights: A teen's boyfriend doesn't

notice she is wearing a new red dress; she thinks that he feels she is ugly, and so tells him she never wants to see him again.

Early Adolescence

Early adolescents are usually 10–13 years old. The transition to adolescence is characterized by puberty. Major developmental issues include:

1. Autonomy: Wide mood swings, desires for privacy.
2. Body image: Critical of appearance and preoccupied with body changes.
3. Peer group: Same sex friendships.
4. Identity: "Am I normal?" Problems often become magnified: "No one understands me."

Cognitive Development

Early adolescents still have *concrete thinking* and have little understanding of consequences. With lack of impulse control and a need for instant gratification, there are more risk-taking behaviors than during childhood. They often set unrealistic vocational goals. They are *focused mostly on the present* and may have little sense of later consequences. As their thinking is still in concrete terms, questions are often answered literally, not abstractly.

Psychosocial Development

Early adolescents start to develop a sense of self and are mostly concerned about themselves, their feelings, thoughts and appearance. Typical *egocentrism* creates a feelings of being "on stage and everybody's watching." They often struggle with shyness, and their sense of right and wrong is concrete and based mostly on rules. Obedience may change to rebelliousness. Early adolescents may experiment with sex and mind-altering drugs, that may result in feelings of anxiety and guilt.

Family, Peers and Community

The hallmark of this stage is the need for *autonomy*. They show a decreased interest in activities with family, and begin to notice or create parental flaws, while accepting less parental advice. The testing of authority creates tension with parents and authority figures. Emotional lability may lead to mood swings, and they may alternate between adult and childish behaviors. Parents are still important role models; input from parents is best if it promotes increasing independence and development of healthy decision-making skills. There is a growing need for more personal privacy. Friendships are often with the same sex. Peer values do not replace those of parents yet. As an emotional void is created with separation from parents, there may be a search for new people to love. There are strong emotional feelings and more feelings of sexual attraction — usually with limited action on these feelings. Many youths drop their membership in supportive youth organizations. Television and radio exert more influence over the adolescent's lifestyle and choices made.

School and Career

Early adolescence requires an adjustment to middle school, often causing social pressures. Grades may drop because of resetting priorities for social life rather than academic work. Since school is the place where norms are communicated, health promotion behaviors can be heavily influenced by school policies and curriculum.

Health Risk and Prevention Activities

Young adolescents may experiment with alcohol, tobacco, and sometimes inhalants. They also suffer an increased risk of head injuries from skateboard and bicycle accidents when not wearing protective helmets. There may ride in vehicles with intoxicated drivers. Boys are more likely than girls to engage in risky behaviors, such as sex, substance use, dangerous recreational vehicle use and other injury-related behaviors. Injuries are the leading cause of death for this age group, and result mostly from motor vehicle and bicycle accidents.

Youths rarely know about the normal variation in the onset and rate of pubertal changes. They need reassurance that they are normal and that their own development is normal. Younger adolescents lack experience and judgment which is difficult to comprehensively train in limited health visits. Provide exploration, support and guidance in health promotion, and discuss opportunities for safe experimentation and healthy autonomy.

Characteristic behaviors of early adolescence

Autonomy

- Challenges authority and family; anti-parent; argumentative and disobedient.
- Feels lonely, has wide mood swings, daydreams.
- Rejects things of childhood.
- Desires more privacy.

Body image
- Preoccupied with physical changes and critical of appearance.
- Anxious about menstruation, wet dreams, masturbation, breast or penis size.

Peer group
- Forms intense friendship with same sex.
- Has contact with opposite sex in groups.

Identity development
- "Am I normal?"
- Changes vocational goals frequently.
- Begins to develop own value system.
- Experiences emerging sexual feelings and sexual exploration.
- Imaginary audience: magnifies own problems; "no one understands."

Middle Adolescence

This group comprises 14- to 17-year-olds. This stage is the *essence of adolescence*, with maximum risk behaviors and a strong peer group influence. Major developmental issues include:

1. Autonomy: Family conflict and emerging independence.
2. Body image: Worried about attractiveness.
3. Peer group: Peers most influential; fads, sexual drives and exploration.
4. Identity: Experimentation and risk behaviors, creative and more capable.

Cognitive Development

Middle adolescents think more abstractly, plan more effectively, and better understand the later consequences of their behaviors. The middle adolescent focuses on making himself/herself more attractive to peers, e.g. changing hair styles or hair color, wearing contact lenses, etc. By middle adolescence, *formal operational thinking* is occurring with an increase in abstract reasoning ability. At times, however, especially when under stress, the middle adolescent may revert to concrete thinking. There is a feeling of omnipotence and immortality, which leads to risk-taking behaviors. There is also increased intellectual ability, creativity and more realistic vocational aspirations.

Psychosocial Development

Middle adolescents sort through values and beliefs to increase the sense of self. Adolescents at this age challenge rules, authority, and struggle with issues of independence.

Conflicts between the values of a cultural group and the society are difficult for minority teens. Emotions are labile at this age, and there may be situational depression. Though they are more comfortable with their sexual identity, those with gender identity issues may experience anxiety, depression, and suicidal ideation.

Family, Peers and Community

Middle adolescents spend less time with their families, with peer group activity dominating over family activity. Challenges to parental control may increase family conflict. Conflicts with parents often increase with the improved ability to comprehend abstract ideas and to use logic and reason, even if faulty. New activities such as driving and dating require negotiation and compromise skills for adapting family rules. Middle adolescents can be very susceptible to peer pressure and are sensitive to the social norms of their peers. Physical and sexual intimacy often occurs at this stage, and teens that drive have more of such opportunities and increased risks. The peer pressure of gangs and neighborhoods can become a maladaptive basis for middle adolescents' behaviors and choices.

School and Career

Middle adolescents in secondary school consider academic decisions that impact future career options. There may be anxiety about academic performance which may also be affected by putting a higher priority on social life. Volunteering and employment provide opportunities to explore vocational interests, but studies suggest that adolescents holding jobs perform less well in academics. Violence in schools is sometimes a problem, and carrying weapons to school poses a very high risk.

Health Risk and Prevention Activities

The norm for middle adolescence is *experimentation*, which can have disastrous results. By their secondary school graduation, 90% of teens in western countries have used alcohol and tried other drugs. At least 20% use cigarettes, and as many as 70% are sexually experienced. This is consistent with the known rates of STDs, unintended pregnancies, and the statistic that 1 in 5 AIDS patients are young adults who acquired the disease during adolescence. Because teens are exposed to so much misinformation from their peers about sexuality, these topics should be systematically clarified by clinicians and educators, even if the teen is sexually experienced.

Positive and negative health-related activities of peers should be evaluated because of their powerful influence. Teens' sense of invincibility suggests there may be a great benefit from a discussion about peer pressure. Family members may need assistance with problem-solving and guidance in negotiating new rules and limits for their teen as they adapt to a changing relationship. Since mid-adolescents' actions and decisions can have lasting effects on the quality of their lives, clinicians and educators should maximally utilize health education techniques, while offering support and guidance to lessen the behavioral health risks of mid-adolescence.

Characteristic behaviors of middle adolescence

Autonomy
- Family conflicts predominate due to ambivalence about emerging independence.

Body image
- Less concern about bodily image, but has increased interest in making themselves more attractive.
- Has excessive physical activity alternating with lethargy.

Peer group
- Strong peer allegiances — fad behavior.
- Sexual drives emerge and begins to explore ability to date and attract a partner.

Identity development
- Experiments with sex, drugs, friends, jobs, risk-taking behaviors.
- Sets more realistic vocational goals. Begins to realize strengths and limitations.
- Has increased intellectual ability and creativity.

Late Adolescence

These 17- to 21-, 22-, 23-, or 24-year-olds are often in college, vocational schools, in the military, or are already working and may be starting families. Major developmental issues include:

1. Autonomy: Taking on adult roles.
2. Body image: Comfortable with body image.
3. Peer group: Relates to individual partners more than to peer group.
4. Identity: Transition to adulthood.

Cognitive Development

Abstract reasoning is established. The ability to compromise is present, and a *conscience* is engaged. There is the ability to delay gratification. Financial independence is closer yet many adolescents who continue with higher education delay this step.

Psychosocial Development

By late adolescence, *formal operational thinking* is achieved with high-level abstract reasoning. Research has shown that parts of the brain responsible for higher level functions are not completely mature until age 25. There are less risk-taking behaviors, but existing ones are often habituated and rationalized with increased intellectual ability.

Family, Peers and Community

The late adolescent revises the relationship with his parents, usually forming a more positive bond. Parental values may be observed in the adolescent's value system. Peer groups become less important, and the adolescent is more comfortable with personal values and his identity. Relationships are less exploitative, and an intimate connection with a selected partner often occurs.

School and Career

Vocational aspirations are clarified as the adolescent enters the military, a parent's business, the job market or higher education. The competition and expenses of higher education can be daunting in many countries.

Health Risk and Prevention Activities

With increased personal abilities and access to adult activities, the young adult who lacks experience and judgment of activities such as driving will benefit from competence evaluation and risk management. There remains risk from DUI and other risk behaviors, but often with more severe consequences. Comprehensive risk screening at this stage is mandatory.

Characteristic behaviors of late adolescence

Autonomy
- Emancipation — to vocational/technical/college and/or work (easy); to adult lifestyle (hard).

Body image
- Usually comfortable with body image.

Peer group
- Decisions/values less influenced by peers.
- Relates to individuals more than to peer groups.
- Selects partner based on individual preference.

Identity development
- Pursues realistic vocational goals with training or actual career employment.
- Relates to family as adult.
- Realizes own limitations and mortality.
- Establishes sexual identity, and sexual activity is more common.
- Establishes ethical and moral value system.
- More capable of intimate, complex relationships. Understands consequences of behavior.

Summary

Adolescence is a developmental *process* with physical, psychological, cognitive, and social changes. Understanding normal pubertal development and its variations precludes inappropriate diagnosis of abnormal development. *Early adolescents* are concrete thinkers with little understanding of the consequences of their actions. *Middle adolescents* have some abstract reasoning but also have beliefs of immortality and omnipotence which encourage risk-taking behaviors. The perspective improves during *late adolescence* with improved abstract reasoning. Every adolescent patient's specific stage of psychosocial developmental requires stage-appropriate evaluation, advice, and health promotion.

An understanding of normal physical and psychosocial development of adolescents is primary to clinical practice and health promotion, and it reassures the patient and parent of normal development. Specific interventions at the appropriate level of psychosocial development can provide *relevant* preventive care and *appropriate* anticipatory guidance. Effective health promotion and disease prevention during adolescence can create a lifetime of good health habits.

Suggested Readings and Bibliography

American Academy of Child and Adolescent Psychiatry. (1999). *Your Adolescent Emotional, Behavioral and Cognitive Development through the Teen Years. What Every Parent Needs to Know: What's Normal, What's Not, and When to Seek Help.* (Harper Collins, USA).

DiMeglio LA, Pescovitz OH. (1997). Disorders of puberty: inactivating and activating molecular mutations. *J Pediatrics*, 131, pp. S8–12.

Kamboj M. (2010). *Handbook of Clinical Pediatrics: An Update for the Ambulatory Pediatrician*, eds. Greydanus, D., Patel D, Reddy V, Feinberg A and Omar, H., Figures 1,2,3 in Chapter 11 "Clinical Issues in Endocrinology," (World Scientific Publishing, Singapore) pp. 206–208.

Marshall WA, Tanner JM. (1969). Variations in pattern of pubertal changes in girls. *Arch Dis Child*, 44, pp. 291–303.

Marshall WA, Tanner JM. (1970). Variations in the pattern of pubertal changes in boys. *Arch Dis Child*, 45, pp. 13–23.

Nathan BM, Palmert MR. (2005). Regulation and disorders of pubertal timing. *Endocrinol Metab Clin North Am*, 34, pp. 617–641.

Plant TM. (2002). Neurophysiology of puberty. *J Adolescent Health*, 31, pp. 185–191.

Rosen DS, Foster C. (2001). Delayed puberty. *Pediatr Rev*, 22, pp. 309–315.

Rosen DS. (2004). Physiologic growth and development during adolescence. *Pediatr Rev*, 25, pp. 194–199.

Styne DM. (1997). New aspects in the diagnosis and treatment of pubertal disorders. *Pediatr Clin North Am*, 44, pp. 505–529.

Tanner JM. (1962). *Growth in Adolescence*, 2nd Edn. (Blackwell Scientific Publications, London).

Suggested Website

Children Now is a non-partisan, independent advocacy voice for children and youth which provides up-to-date information on the status of children and youth; as well as outreach to parents, lawmakers, citizens, business, media and community leaders. This site provides information for parents about "talking with kids about tough issues," fact sheets on a variety of child and teen health and health care delivery issues, and an annotated publications list including a series on the effects of television: http://www.childrennow.org

Chapter 3

Dermatology

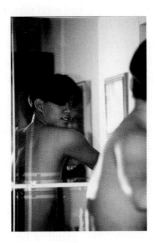

Overview

Skin lesions and conditions, including acne, represent a significant number of visits to primary care providers, and offer a frequent opportunity to establish immediate and effective rapport with adolescent patients in order to also accomplish health risk screening and health promotion. It is common for adolescents to self-treat numerous skin conditions, some of which may have significant morbidity.

Acne

Acne is a problem for nearly all adolescents, with a high incidence count of about 85%. Adolescents are normally self-conscious about their appearance, so acne can be very distressing. Acne can cause lowered self-esteem and social withdrawal. Unfortunately, relatively few adolescents see a clinician for treatment, instead using over-the-counter preparations that are aggressively marketed to a vulnerable audience. Primary care providers can treat nearly all teenagers with acne, except the most severe cases. Only a few basic medications are used, but counseling and guidance about acne care needs to be effective in order to facilitate compliance in spite of usual impatience.

A 17-year-old female presented to the office with a history of using an "acne wash and cream" that was recommended by a clinician last year which she stopped using because it made her acne worse and burned her face. Now, she irregularly uses an over-the-counter acne soap, and puts on a cream at night that she ordered on the Internet. With fair skin, her face had mild papulopustular acne with a few comedones, while her back had no acne. She was informed that the proposed treatment will result in some facial dryness, which she can expect, along with worsening of the acne before any improvement is observed. However, because of past sensitivity to drying agents, she is to start with 5% benzoyl peroxide wash twice a day, followed by 5% benzoyl peroxide gel combined with a topical antibiotic. She was told to call the office if problems arise, but not to stop treatment or use other medications, soaps, or treatments. After 1 month, she is to switch to 10% benzoyl peroxide wash as tolerated, and a month after that to 10% benzoyl peroxide gel combined with the topical antibiotic. She faithfully carried out the twice-a-day routine, returned monthly for follow-ups, and was pleased with her results.

Acne is caused by the pilosebaceous gland, a blocked hair follicle which can become inflamed and lead to scarring. Males generally have worse acne than females because of higher androgen levels. There is a genetic familial predisposition. With androgenic stimulation, sebaceous glands produce more sebum in the follicle. Androgens enlarge the sebaceous glands and also increase the bacteria, *Proprionibacterium acnes*, which is normally found in the skin. Androgenic oral contraceptives can worsen acne. Oil-based cosmetics can further block follicles. No foods have ever been proven to cause or worsen acne (in spite of many anecdotes), but stress probably exacerbates acne, and of course, acne causes more stress.

There are two categories of lesions:

1. Non-inflammatory: comedones, papules.
2. Inflammatory: pustules, nodules, cysts, and (resulting) scars.

Papulopustular is the common description of transitional acne with both features.

Medications

The drying action of many medications is a major cause of non-compliance. Gels are more drying and irritating because they penetrate more than creams and lotions, but they are often well tolerated. *Benzoyl peroxide* is the primary and initial treatment, and after 5 days of use (twice a day), it will eliminate nearly all of *P. acnes*. A 2.5% gel is more effective than the 10% lotion, and the 2.5% gel is as effective as the 10% gel against *P. acnes*, but is less drying and irritating. Benzoyl peroxide is often combined with topical *clindamycin* or *erythromycin* in mixed preparations for those who are non-compliant or have drying and irritated skin. Benzoyl peroxide should not be applied immediately after washing the face, since moisture increases absorption, and it should not be used with other medicines unless it is a mixed preparation. Always begin with a simple treatment plan, and give adolescents a choice of treatment approaches if possible.

Normally, benzoyl peroxide needs to be used twice a day before assessing the results. Treatment of acne often requires progressively stronger medications with regular reevaluation for every increase in strength. To avoid initial irritation, often start with a 5% lotion or gel once a day. After 1 week, increase use to twice a day (morning and night) if the skin is not too irritated. After 6 more weeks, increase to a 10% strength lotion or gel, starting with one application each day, then two daily applications as tolerated. Patients need to be warned that treatment may require some worsening of the acne before improvement. Washing of the face and applying medication must eventually be twice a day. Patients should be told not to stop treatment or use other medications, soaps, or treatments. If ever there is too much dryness or irritation, patients can decrease the frequency of use of the gel or cream, and later work back up to twice a day as tolerated. Patients should also be warned about the potential staining of clothing and towels.

Often benzoyl peroxide is used in the morning while *Retin-A* is used in the evening. Retin-A cream or gel helps unplug oil ducts, and is best for comedones, yet patients often feel their acne worsening before improving. It may take months for complete results. Patients should let their face dry before application and also be aware that exposure to the sun can cause increased redness in skin. Differin is a newer retinoid which is less irritating than Retin-A.

Topical antibiotic solutions of clindamycin or erythromycin are used in combination with other medications, particularly for pustular acne and in mitigation of dryness and irritation. When used consistently, they are as effective as their oral preparations. Oral antibiotics such as tetracycline may be used if the acne does not respond adequately to topical treatments. Tetracycline is better tolerated orally than erythromycin and is safer than clindamycin. The side effect of candidal vaginitis is more common than erythema multiforme or pseudotumor cerebri.

For females, estrogenic oral contraceptives such as Demulen or Ortho Tri-Cyclen can assist in the treatment of moderate to severe acne (and can also serve as a reason for parents as to why their child is on an oral contraceptive). For males, isotretinoin (Accutane) is used only for severe cystic acne that has not responded to other treatments. For females, it has potentially serious side effects and must never be used in those who may become pregnant. It must be discontinued at least 1 month before a woman becomes pregnant. Patients who take Accutane must be carefully supervised by a doctor knowledgeable about its use, and who can also address sexual behaviors.

Counseling Items for Adolescent Acne Patients

- Be patient — give each treatment enough time to work.
- Be faithful — follow your treatment plan every day. Do not stop and start each time your skin changes.
- Remember — sometimes your skin may appear to worsen early in the program before you begin to see improvement.
- Follow directions — not using the treatment as directed is the most common reason the treatment fails.
- Do not overdo it — more is not better. Too much scrubbing makes skin worse. Too much benzoyl peroxide or Retin-A cream makes your skin red and scaly.
- Oral antibiotics may suppress symptoms of STDs, may have a variety of side effects, and improper use may cause resistant organisms.

Common Conditions

Only the more common dermatologic conditions affecting adolescents will be discussed here. Sexually transmitted infections discussed in Chapter 7 also cause both widespread and localized dermatologic findings.

Dermatitis

Contact dermatitis is an allergic reaction of the skin to a specific allergen, often making the contact area itchy, dry and scaly. It usually makes the skin irritated and the skin loses its protective barriers. Metal jewelry and plant saps are common causes. Daily measures to prevent skin damage include:

- Using soaps and detergents which minimize damage to the skin's protective oils, and using moisturizers to reinforce the skin's protective oils.
- Recommend Dove, Aveno or Neutrogena, cleansers instead of soap, and moisturizers such as Lubriderm, Keri, Moisturel or Eucerin.

- Keep the skin covered to prevent scratching, especially at night.
- Keep fingernails short and clean to reduce infection.
- To treat rash flare ups, use hydrocortisone, desonide, or triamcinolone cream or ointment twice a day for a week or more. Benadryl may be used at bedtime to reduce itching and scratching.

Atopic dermatitis (eczema) is a long-lasting (chronic) allergic skin condition that is itchy, dry and scaly. It is controllable but generally not curable, nor contagious. A sensitive immune system reacts to irritants and allergens which should be avoided. Again, prevention is by use of non-drying cleansers (Dove, Aveno, Neutrogena) and moisturizers (Lubriderm, Keri, Moisturel, Eucerin, Cetaphil). Fingernails must be kept short and clean to reduce infection. Medication for eczema flare ups include: Hydrocortisone, desonide, or triamcinolone cream or ointment for weeks. If severe, then daily prevention may involve Protopic ointment or generous use of Cetaphil or Vaseline. Oral antihistamines such as diphenhydramine (Benadryl) or chlorpheniramine (Chlor-Trimeton) are especially useful at bedtime to reduce itching and scratching. Minor bacterial infections can usually be treated with antibiotic ointments, but oral antibiotics are sometimes necessary for more extensive infections.

Seborrhea/dandruff is a common, scaly, crusty rash of the scalp. Crusting is formed by skin oils and the dead skin cells that normally fall off, along with an allergic reaction. To treat dandruff, anti-dandruff shampoos such as Head and Shoulders, Selsun Blue or T-gel are used. Patients must rub it in and leave it on for an adequate amount of time for effectiveness.

Pityriasis alba is a condition of the skin that is often found in atopic individuals that makes the skin dry and scaly. One theory is that the involved areas have thicker stratum corneum layers and thus allow less sun in and hence, less pigmentation. Like a mild form of eczema, especially seen on the face in dark complexions, it is often called "sun spots" as it appears to get worse with sun exposure and drying of skin. The appearance is caused by the normal surrounding skin getting darker, while the affected skin remains light. It can be prevented by moisturizing the skin regularly (Lubriderm, Keri, Moisturel, Eucerin, Cetaphil) and by using non-drying cleansers (Dove, Aveno, Neutrogena). Medications include hydrocortisone or Desonide cream or ointment.

Vectors

Insect bites cause swelling from the body's reaction to the insect saliva. Swelling is often large, puffy, pinkish, and itchy. If the insect bite is found near the eye, it can even swell closed. Insect bites generally do not get infected, and do not require antibiotics, but when finally seen by a clinician, they may have some component of infection when they appear deeply red, more swollen, hard (vs. puffy), and painful when touched.

Prevent mosquito bites by reducing their breeding areas. They breed in standing water, and they do not travel more than 200 yards from their birthplace. Patients should check living areas for standing water and clear it, including buckets, flower pots, old tires and other small amounts of standing water. Long-sleeved shirts and pants help prevent bites in mosquito-prone areas. To repel mosquitoes, various sprays, pads and lotions are available. Permethrin spray is safe to spray on clothing, tents, and mosquito nets, and is available without prescription. To treat bites, an oral antihistamine is the best approach. Diphenhydramine at bedtime and Loratadine (non-drowsy) in the morning is a good combination. Calamine applied topically may or may not help reduce severe itching. Remind patients to return to the clinic if the bite becomes red, more swollen, hard, or sore.

Scabies is a pruritic dermatitis that is caused by the itch mite which burrows into the skin. It is acquired from people and pets that carry the mite. They rarely affect the skin above the neck. Common medicines include Permethrin 5% or Crotamiton 10% cream of which is applied to the entire body overnight and washed off in the morning. Bed sheets and the patient's clothes should be washed in hot water. If the rash does not respond in 2 weeks, or if it gets worse, reevaluate it. The patient may need medications for itching such as Diphenhydramine at bedtime. Topical steroids may suppress the itch but are not recommended since they may allow fulminant scabies to spread.

Head lice, acquired from other people and pets that carry the louse, lay eggs on the hair. Medicated shampoos such as RID should stay in the hair for 10 minutes before rinsing. Repeat the treatment in 1 week, and comb the hair with a fine comb to remove the nits. The dead nits do not have to be removed, however. In hot water, wash bed sheets, the patient's clothes, any hats or other materials that come into contact with the hair. If the rash does not respond in 2 weeks, or if it gets worse, reevaluate it.

Bacterial Infections

Impetigo is a bacterial infection of the skin, often caused by *Staphylococcus* or *Streptococcus*. The patient should wash the skin well with soap and water, cut the fingernails, and keep the wounds covered to prevent spread. Hot soaks with a strong antiseptic such as Betadine (povidone iodine 10% solution) can help eliminate many skin infections. They often require oral antibiotics if severe, widespread or if found on the face. Cellulitis is a deeper bacterial infection where the skin is hard, warm, tender and red, often with a well-defined edge. Since this can spread rapidly, oral or parenteral antibiotics as well as applications of heat are usually indicated.

A 22-year-old male has a 5-day history of a "sore on the left arm with pus" which he had squeezed, and it worsened shortly thereafter. He took a few leftover pills of his sister's antibiotics, and now redness is spreading. Upon examination of the left forearm, there is a 5 cm area of warm erythema with a centrally indurated area, slightly draining a yellow discharge. A sample of the drainage was taken for culture and sensitivity. The patient was warned about taking leftover antibiotics, and was started on oral amoxicillin-clavulanate for cellulitis with draining abscess, and was instructed not to squeeze the lesion, but to apply hot compresses of half-strength Betadine approximately 1 hour after taking the medication twice a day. On return to the clinic in 2 days, the lesion was only slightly improved, and there was a new impetigo at the right nostril. Previous culture revealed methicillin-resistant *Staphylococcus aureus* which was resistant to amoxicillin-clavulanate and sensitive to ceftriaxone, trimethoprim-sulfasoxazole and vancomycin. The patient was given intramuscular ceftriaxone, switched to oral trimethoprim-sulfasoxazole, and warned about infection spread to family members. He kept his fingernails short and clean, applied antibiotic ointment to the nares, and both lesions resolved in the next few days.

Methicillin-resistant *Staphylococcus aureus* (MRSA) can be resistant to many antibiotics. The bacteria are widespread on the skin and in the nose, and it can cause infections of the skin, heart, blood, and bones. Treat with antibiotics of known community sensitivity, and always do cultures and sensitivity testing. Often, vancomycin or other antibiotics may be necessary. Use Betadine locally in combination with an antibiotic ointment on lesions, and use antibiotic ointment in the nose. Patients should avoid contact with others while infected. Counseling emphasis should be made about follow-up care as an important part of treatment, not missing suggested appointments, taking antibiotics exactly as directed and watching for signs of problems.

Information for Patients with Bacterial Skin Infections

- Do not stop taking antibiotics just because you feel better. You need to take the full course of antibiotics.
- Keep any cuts or other wounds covered while they heal.
- Wash your hands often, especially after touching elastic bandages or other dressings over a wound. This can keep the bacteria from spreading. Wrap bandages in a plastic bag before you throw them away.
- Do not share towels, washcloths, razors, clothing, or other items that touched your wound or bandage.

Viral Infections

There are numerous rashes and signs of viral infection manifested by the skin, some of which like herpesvirus are discussed in Chapter 7, but only a few of the more common ones are discussed here.

Hives (Urticaria) is a common allergic disorder. It can be caused by a virus or by an allergy. An allergy is often to foods or medicines. Often, the etiology remains unknown. If it persists for more than 2 weeks or recurs frequently, a workup may include CBC, differential, and stool for ova and parasites. Acute hives are very itchy and usually require oral antihistamines.

Varicella zoster (shingles) is usually a relatively benign varicella infection of the skin that occurs years after chickenpox infection. Vesicles are usually found in a single band across the chest along a dermatome or along nerve branches on one side of the body. The chickenpox virus can be dormant for 30 or 40 years in nerve roots, but lesions do occur in various areas. It is quite painful and can be debilitating. Preceding the blisters for several days, there may only be pain which is often understandably mistaken for chest pain or myalgia. The rash will resolve in about 1 week without treatment in most cases, however, some scarring can occur in those who are prone to scars. Sometimes, it leaves residual scars when the infection has been severe or if secondary bacterial infection developed. Adults may get "lingering neuralgia" in the healed area for many months or even years.

Since it can transmit chickenpox to people who are susceptible, the rash should be covered until all of the lesions are crusted over. Treatment includes oral antihistamine for itching, as well as soothing baths in oatmeal bath suspension or Aveno. An anti-septic soap can reduce the chances of developing secondary bacterial infection; calamine lotion may help. Other medications to reduce the symptoms include acetaminophen to relieve the burning, and zinc oxide ointment is also useful. Oral Acyclovir is used in severe cases, particularly if lesions are affecting the eye or face. There can be scarring of the eye with possible partial loss of vision, so eye infections are usually followed by an ophthalmologist.

Pityriasis rosea is a benign skin condition found commonly in teens. The exact cause is unknown, but it is probably caused by a harmless virus, since it seems to appear in epidemic clusters. This rash often begins on the torso in a large patch called a herald patch. A mildly pruritic, rosey rash then appears up to 3 weeks after the herald patch, and progresses for 10–14 days. It can last 3 months, which distresses most adolescent patients. This rash will resolve without complications or any treatment. It is rarely accompanied by a mild fever, malaise, headache, or achy joints. Moisturizers and oral antihistamine medications can help alleviate itch, but do not cure the condition. Mild sun exposure may help, with care not to allow sunburn.

Warts are non-malignant skin growths caused by human papilloma virus infection in the skin. They are most common where skin has been broken. Plantar warts on the soles of the feet rise above the skin surface due to pressure and can be painful. Flat warts are small and smooth and there can be large numbers in an area. Warts grow slowly — often several months before becoming symptomatic. The contagiousness of hand, foot, or flat warts from person to person is small. The wart virus enters more easily if the skin has been damaged, like punctures on the sole of the foot. Adolescents with weak immune systems also tend to have warts. Warts may disappear without treatment over several months or years. Salicylic acid gel, solution, or plaster may need to be used for many weeks of treatment. Cryotherapy and application of other medicines may be useful, as well as many surgical treatments. On the feet, adolescents should use foot pads to reduce pressure on the wart, and keep the feet dry, since moisture tends to allow warts to spread.

Fungal Infections

Tinea versicolor is a harmless superficial fungus, *Malassezia furfur*. It favors persons who have oily skin with abundant perspiration and who lack inherited immunity to mold growth. It occurs most frequently in warm, humid tropical climates and most commonly affects the neck, shoulders, chest, and upper arms. More extensive involvement includes the scalp hairline, lower face, lower arms, waistline, abdomen, buttocks, groin, and upper thighs. The color varies from whitish to light pink, but it is usually fawn (beige) colored. Versicolor refers to this variability of color. On sun-tanned skin, the mold appears pale white, whereas on pale skin the mold appears fawn colored. Most persons diagnose it themselves before they see a doctor. However, in less typical cases, diagnosis can be confirmed by examination of a scraping of the scales under a microscope or observance of a characteristic "golden yellow fluorescence" of the scales when viewed with an ultraviolet lamp (Woods Light) in a darkened room.

There are two stages:
1. The fawn-colored stage is beige or light brown irregular fine-scaly spots.
2. The white-colored stage is where the skin under the mold spots loses its pigments as the sun is progressively screened out by the mold, producing a gradual change from fawn to white colored.

About 1 in 10 adolescents in tropical climates develops this mold, related to immunity, climate, sweat, and skin oil. It is only mildly contagious, depending on individual susceptibility (lack of immunity). Husband and wife may sleep together for years and yet only one of them may have it.

One treatment is: Every night for a week, gently run a scrub sponge over affected areas, then lather Selsun Blue or Exsel shampoo into the wet skin for 5 minutes and then shower off. Later, apply a half-strength dilution of this shampoo to stay on the skin all night. Repeat treatment one night weekly for 1 month. Selenium sulphide contained in Selsun or Exsel kills the fungus on the skin. Alternatively, Tinver lotion, Micatin, Spectazole, Lotrimin or Mycelex cream or lotion are used. Additional measures to reduce recurrences include showering with a sulfur soap. During treatment, wash bed linen, towels, and underclothes weekly in hot water containing a bleach disinfectant, followed by hot ironing to kill any residual fungus spores. During the treatment period and thereafter, exposure to the sun is desirable to speed up repigmentation of the white spots left under the original mold. Return of the white spots to normal tan color may take as long as a year, depending on how much time is spent in sun exposure.

Tinea cruris may appear on one or both sides of the groin as a slowly progressive itchy rash with an advancing reddish border and a scaling, clearing center. It commonly spreads to the pubic region or the inner surfaces of the legs or buttocks. (Usually there is no spread to the scrotum, where the skin is thin.) Sometimes the rash will begin on the buttocks. It can be spread by contact with contaminated objects such as locker room benches and floors, gymnastic equipment, swimming pool lounge chairs, wearing someone else's swimwear, as well as by sexual relations.

Fungal infection of the skin is a cosmetic nuisance, tends to itch and is socially embarrassing. About 75% of the world has natural hereditary immunity, but the remaining 25% lacking this are susceptible to a lifetime of repeated occurrences. Youths in poor health tend to have lowered resistance to fungus. Those with diabetes are more prone to fungal infections, just as they are more prone to bacterial infections and slow healing.

The usual treatment is an antifungal cream or lotion applied twice a day for 3 weeks. Though it may appear clear in 1 or 2 weeks, patients should treat the area for an additional week to prevent recurrence from residual dormant spores in the hair follicles. When the fungus is of a longer duration (a few months) and involves a wider area, it is sometimes necessary to treat the fungus with oral medication (like Lamasil or griseofulvin) in addition to the antifungal cream or lotion. These medications may have side effects that should be monitored.

Tinea corporis or ringworm is a similar fungal infection which exhibits a scaly red patch. This is usually in the shape of a ring, and enlarges with clearing in the center. It is similarly treated with an antifungal cream or lotion.

Tinea capitus is a fungal infection of the scalp which sometimes causes a bald spot and/or dandruff. The suggested treatment is selenium sulfide shampoo two times a week or more often. Usually, topical treatment alone is not effective for tinea capitus due to the involvement of the fungus deep within the follicles, so this condition is usually treated with an oral antifungal medicine.

Sun Exposure and Skin Cancer

Sun exposure and suntans cause premature aging of skin, and repeated sunburns increase skin cancer risk — in fact, *each blistering sunburn doubles the risk of melanoma.* To prevent skin cancer, prevent sunburn. Skin cancer occurs in adulthood, but it is caused by cumulative sun exposure and burns during childhood and adolescence.

Sunscreen

Sunscreen in adolescence prevents skin cancer later. Some sunscreens prevent sunburn but permit gradual tanning. Do not recommend suntan lotions or oil that only lubricate the skin. A sunscreen with sun protection factor (SPF) of 15 allows only 7% of the sun's rays to penetrate and extends safe sun exposure from a half hour to 5 hours. SPFs of over 30 may not dramatically improve sun protection, but they can be helpful for sun-sensitive individuals (due to medications, skin color, medical conditions like lupus) and can be helpful if a lower SPF sunscreen is not applied thoroughly. However, if applied correctly and frequently enough, anything above SPF 30 may not be very cost effective.

Sunscreen should be used for every exposure of 30 minutes or more. It should be applied generously and *repeatedly.* Most people apply too little and do not reapply every few hours. Opaque zinc oxide ointment protects the nose best. Adolescents should avoid sun exposure between 10 a.m. and 3 p.m., during the most intense sunlight. About a third of the sun's rays penetrate common woven fabrics and T-shirts. Water, sand, and snow increase sun exposure by reflection. Since skin cancer often occurs on the face, recommend caps or hats. Fair-skinned adolescents who do not tan but burn are at very high risk, especially those with red or blond hair, blue or green eyes, or freckles. Protect the eyes with ultraviolet (UV) protective sunglasses since exposure to ultraviolet light increases the risk of getting cataract at a later age.

Sunburn

Sunburn caused by exposure of the skin to UV rays has symptoms that often do not begin for 3 or 4 hours. Maximum redness, pain, and swelling occurs about 24 hours later. Mild sunburn is a first-degree burn with redness. Blistering is a second-degree burn. Sunburn does not cause third-degree burns. Treatment of minor sunburn includes ibuprofen started early (taken for 2 days), and hydrocortisone cream which should be used early. Blisters that open should be covered with antibiotic ointment. The use of cool baths and cool, wet compresses help relieve pain and burning. Extra fluids are necessary to replace fluid loss in tissues. Peeling usually occurs in about a week, and dry skin should not be peeled before the skin underneath is completely healed. Use moisturizing creams. A short course of oral prednisone has been used in severe cases.

Melanoma and Nevi

Malignant melanoma is the most deadly of all skin cancers. It starts in melanocytes, the skin cells that produce melanin. Since melanoma cells usually continue to produce melanin, lesions can appear in mixed shades of tan, brown, and black, although they can also be red or white. Since melanoma is often lethal when it metastasizes, early detection and treatment are essential, particularly for those adolescents who may have had a number of blistering sunburns as a child. Lesions may appear suddenly or begin in or near a mole or other dark spot in the skin. It is important for adolescents to know the location and appearance of their moles to be able to detect changes early.

There is increased risk of melanoma if a relative or close family member has had a history of melanoma. Having atypical moles, which may run in families, and having a large number of moles are markers for people at increased risk. Most moles are harmless. However, pre-cancerous moles should be promptly excised. The most damage by sun exposure has occurred by age 20, so counsel younger adolescents that cumulative exposure to sun is a major contributing factor in later skin cancer.

Warning Signs of Melanoma
• Changes in the surface of a mole.
• Scaliness, oozing, bleeding, or the appearance of a new bump.
• Spread of pigment from the border of a mole into surrounding skin.
• Change in sensation including itchiness, tenderness, or pain.

Identifying Melanoma

Normal moles are brown, tan, or black spots. They may be flat or raised, with sharply-defined borders. Most moles are harmless, but patients must watch for changes as well as "moles" that are abnormal in shape, color, or diameter. A melanoma can appear flat or raised with irregular edges. Its color can vary from red to black. It may bleed easily. The sudden appearance of a new mole in or near an existing mole, or a mole that has changed shape or color, should be considered suspicious. Adolescents should check their skin regularly for changes or new lesions.

ABCDE: Characteristics of Atypical Nevi or Melanoma
- A = Asymmetry — one half of a mole does not match the other.
- B = Border irregularity — the edges are ragged, notched or blurred.
- C = Color — the color varies from one area to another, with shades of tan and brown, black, or sometimes white, red or blue.
- D = Diameter — larger than a 6 mm circle (a pencil eraser).
- E = Enlargement — any enlargement of a mole.

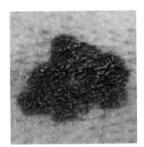 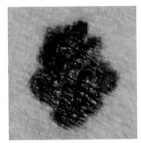 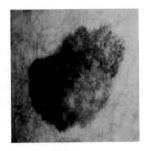

Patients should examine the skin with a mirror, looking for unusual moles, spots, or bumps, paying special attention to areas that receive a lot of sun exposure — hands, arms, chest, neck (especially the back), face, and ears. If moles do not change over time, there is little cause for concern. It is useful to take annual digital photos of every mole on the body with a nearby coin for sizing. If there is a family history of malignant melanoma, an annual examination and health education is advisable.

Tattoos and Body Piercing

Adolescents often get tattoos or body parts pierced because they like body art or like to express themselves. Some get a tattoo or piercing to feel like part of a group. In some jurisdictions, they need to be age 18 or have their parent's permission to legally get a piercing or tattoo. Adolescents should be informed about the possible health risks. If they do decide to have a tattoo or body piercing, it is important that it is done safely. Teenagers sometimes make decisions about tattoos and body piercing when they are emotionally upset. They should wait until they have had time to think carefully about it before making this decision.

Tattoos are injected into the skin with a tattoo machine. Most people say it is a painful process. If an adolescent later becomes unhappy with a tattoo or regrets getting it, it is a painful and very expensive process to try to remove it. Tattoos should be considered permanent. Removing a tattoo, even a small one, is not only expensive but usually leaves a scar. Many young adults who get a tattoo later regret doing so because they are embarrassed by the design or location of the tattoo. Furthermore, a tattoo can make it more difficult to get a job. Counsel that it is advisable to wear a temporary tattoo before making a final decision.

Body piercing is a hole made in the skin with a hollow needle. The body jewelry is then inserted into the hole. Such jewelry should be made of surgical stainless steel, or 14- or 18-karat gold, niobium, or titanium. It should not contain nickel because it is known to cause allergic reactions. Jewelry should be the right fit for the body part pierced. Piercing guns should never be used because they cannot be properly sterilized. Piercing navels is not recommended due to the incidence of infection.

Only a professional tattoo or body-piercing artist should do such work. Adolescents should never tattoo or pierce themselves or friends. The risk of infection and other complications is greater when they apply their own body art. Patients must beware of a tattoo or piercing parlor that is willing to bend the rules about age of consent. Carefully investigate the establishment where tattooing or piercing may be done. Only new, sterilized needles should be used. Tattoos and body piercing can cause bacterial infection. Many viral infections can be spread during the process of getting body art. Tattooing and body piercing can also cause allergic reactions. Some people have an allergy to the pigments used in tattoos or the metals in jewelry. Again, choose jewelry made of stainless steel, titanium, or 14-karat gold, and avoid jewelry that may contain nickel. The following symptoms may need medical treatment: redness, warmth, tenderness, or swelling that is excessive or that lasts longer than a few days, yellow or green discharge or pus, or oozing or bleeding that lasts longer than several days.

Some Risks of Tattooing and Body Piercing

- Bleeding.
- Scars, including large keloids, especially on ears.
- Bacterial skin infections.
- Haemophilus aphrophilus endocarditis after tongue piercing.
- Allergic reactions to dyes and metals (pigments are typically not regulated by government.)
- Hepatitis B and C, HIV/AIDS, and tetanus (complete series of Hepatitis B and tetanus vaccines help reduce risk.)
- Torn skin like a ripped earlobe (visible jewelry and tongue studs should be removed before participation in sports to avoid injury.)
- Chipping of teeth and speech problems caused by tongue and lip rings.

Suggested Readings and Bibliography

American Academy of Dermatology. (2010). Melanoma Trends. Available from: http://www. aad.org/media/background/factsheets/fact_melanomatrends.html.

American Academy of Dermatology. (2010). Melanoma Fact Sheet. Available from: http://www. aad.org/media/background/factsheets/fact_melanoma.html.

Bone A, Ncube F, Nichols T, Noah ND. (2008). Body piercing in England: a survey of piercing at sites other than earlobe. *BMJ*, 336, pp. 1426–1428.

Braverman PK. (2006). Body art: piercing, tattooing, and scarification. *Adolesc Med Clin*, 17, pp. 505–519.

Buchanan N, Leisenring W, Mitby PA, *et al.* (2009). Behaviors associated with ultraviolet radiation exposure in a cohort of adult survivors of childhood and adolescent cancer: a report from the Childhood Cancer Survivor Study. *Cancer*, 115, pp. 4374–4384.

Carroll ST, Riffenburgh RH, Roberts TA, *et al.* (2002). Tattoos and body piercings as indicators of adolescent risk-taking behaviors. *Pediatrics*, 109, pp.1021–1027.

Cho H, Sands LP, Wilson KM. (2010). Predictors of summer sun safety practice intentions among rural high school students. *Am J Health Behav*, 34, pp. 412–419.

Dennis LK, Vanbeek MJ, Beane Freeman LE, *et al.* (2008). Sunburns and risk of cutaneous melanoma: does age matter? A comprehensive meta-analysis. *Ann Epidemiol*, 18, pp. 614–627.

Gollnick H, Cunliffe W, Berson D, *et al.* (2003). Management of acne: a report from a Global Alliance to Improve Outcomes in Acne. *J Am Acad Dermatol*, 49, pp. S1–37.

Hofmann AD, Greydanus DE (eds). (1997). Chapter 18 in *Adolescent Medicine*. 3rd Edn. (McGraw-Hill/Appleton & Lange, USA). ISBN-13: 978-0838500675.

Houghton SJ, Durkin K, Parry E, *et al.* (1996). Amateur tattooing practices and beliefs among high school adolescents. *J Adolesc Health*, 19, pp. 420-425.

Krowchuk DP. (2005). Managing adolescent acne: a guide for pediatricians. *Pediatr Rev*, 26, pp. 250–261.

Mayers LB, Chiffriller SH. (2008). Body art (body piercing and tattooing) among undergraduate university students: "then and now." *J Adolesc Health*, 42, pp. 201–203.

Navarro DS. (2008) What teens should know about oral piercings. *School Nurse News*, 25, pp. 25–26.

Quéreux G, Nguyen JM, Volteau C, *et al.* (2010). Creation and test of a questionnaire for self-assessment of melanoma risk factors. *Eur J Cancer Prev*, 19, pp. 48–54.

Roberts TA, Ryan SA. (2002). Tattooing and high-risk behavior in adolescents. *Pediatrics*, 110, pp. 1058–1063.

Thieden E. (2009). Sun protection in teenagers. *BMJ*, 338: a2997.

Suggested Websites

American Academy of Dermatology: http://www.aad.org

American Cancer Society: http://www.cancer.org

Chapter 4

Chronic Disease Management

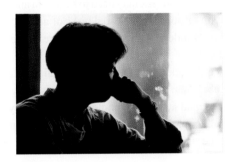

On SUCCESS –
to laugh often and much
to win respect of intelligent people and the affection of children,
to earn the appreciation of honest critics and endure the betrayal of false
friends,
to appreciate beauty,
to find the best in others,
to leave the world a bit better, whether by a healthy child, a garden patch
or a redeemed social condition,
to know even one life has breathed easier because you have lived.
This is to have succeeded. —Ralph Waldo Emerson

Overview

Adolescents with chronic handicapping conditions (CHC) or developmental disabilities (DD) should participate in decision making regarding their care, school-
ing, and future. They must still be provided opportunities for recreation, education,

transportation, and employment. If limitations prevent participation in the same manner as other teens and young adults, then physical and social accommodations must be made. Chronic medical conditions (CMC) such as asthma, diabetes, eating disorders, constipation, and chronic pain, interfere with the lives and lifestyles of adolescents and young adults, sometimes to the extent that they can become physically and emotionally handicapping conditions.

Concerns about body image may be magnified depending on the condition or disability. While developmental tasks are the same for all adolescents, they may occur out of sequence for youths with CHC and DD. An adolescent may be emotionally ready for independence from the family, but physical difficulties may interfere with the degree of independence he or she is able to achieve at that time. An example for DD might be sexuality issues where interest in sex may peak, while socially acceptable ways of dealing with feelings about sex may need to be taught and monitored. Similarly, CMCs often interfere with or obstruct the usual tasks of adolescents. Separation from the family and the desire for independence are often more challenging for adolescents with CMC, CHC or DD.

It is important to see the adolescent as an individual first, and to be sensitive to the use of a "label". Labels can unlock doors to services, provide access to support systems, or contribute to equal access accommodations, but they also can obscure the individual behind them. "People first" language is a way of saying that you respect the person first (e.g. a teenager with diabetes, a youth who is blind, or an adolescent with asthma).

Parents of adolescents with CMC, CHC or DD share the same concerns as parents of other adolescents. Anxiety may be heightened within some families with regard to medical fragility, safety, communication, independent living, medical care in the adult system, decision making, sexuality, and employment.

Medical Compliance and Self-Management

Adolescent compliance with medical regimens and advice requires the patient to feel that the physician really cares about him or her. A clear and coordinated treatment plan is important, but in spite of our best efforts, the processes of *avoidance* and *denial* are often a significant part of the psychology of adolescents regarding their chronic medical conditions: "If I just ignore this diabetes, it may go away."; "I'm just coughing a little; it's not a big asthma attack."; "It's too hard to change my diet; I get constipated anyway."

The use of complimentary and alternative medicine (CAM) and dietary supplements among adolescents are increasing and remain largely unregulated. The former may exclude necessary and effective medical care, and the latter may have potentially negative side effects. In westernized countries, about three-quarters of adolescents have tried a CAM, and half used one in the last month. About half of adolescents have ever used a dietary supplement, and a third used one in the last month. Common supplements among adolescents include zinc, echinacea, weight loss supplements and creatine — the latter two are linked with attempts to change body shape. Clinicians must include CAM and dietary supplements in the medical history and evaluate incompatibilities with concurrent treatment plans and prescription medications.

Self-Esteem and Compliance

Self-esteem is intimately tied to one's ability and willingness to engage in self-management of medical conditions. Self-esteem is often defined as the way a person feels about him- or herself, but it is also a personal view of one's capability to accomplish goals, such as self-management of disease. Conversely, having a disease requiring ongoing care can affect the personal view of one's capability to manage their lives.

A Person with High Self-Esteem
- Is proud of their accomplishments.
- Acts independently.
- Assumes responsibility.
- Tolerates frustration.
- Approaches new challenges with enthusiasm.
- Feels capable of influencing their peers.
- Is usually capable of managing their chronic disease.

A Person with Low Self-Esteem
- Avoids situations that stimulate fear or anxiety.
- Demeans their own talents.
- Feels unliked and unwanted.
- Is overly influenced by others.
- Becomes easily frustrated.
- Feels powerless.
- Is often incapable of managing their chronic disease.

According to Reynold Bean [Bean, 1992], self-esteem is a state that results from four senses of being. These are found within the individual and in his or her environment — a sense of uniqueness, connectedness, power, and models. To help an adolescent develop and build self-esteem, address the follow:

1. Know who you are — identify strengths and weaknesses.
2. Take a look at what makes you feel good and bad about yourself.
3. Identify people in your life who are builders and who are blockers.
4. Identify things in your life that are builders and that are blockers.
5. Explore what you know and have learned about yourself.

Decision Making and Goal Setting

If personal problems and issues are not carefully considered, the consequences can have far reaching effects on future health decisions. Adolescents need to have an understanding about decision making and the steps they can use to make good decisions about managing their health conditions. Knowing these steps will help to increase adolescents' sense of control over their lives and enable them to accept responsibility for the decisions they do make. Making good decisions that impact their life in a positive way will increase self-esteem. When the need arises to make a health decision, there are six important steps.

Health Decision Making Process
1. Determine if there is a decision to be made; describe it out loud.
2. Examine the choices.
3. Collect information and identify other influences on the decision.
4. Investigate the consequences of choices.
5. Decide which action is responsible, optimal and most appropriate.
6. Evaluate the results of the decision.

Enabling adolescents to make good decisions will empower them to effectively handle chronic health conditions. Accomplishing goals plays a major role in developing self-esteem. Goals need to be realistic and well planned. There are six characteristics of realistic health goals.

Realistic Health Goals
1. Definable
2. Desirable
3. Attainable
4. Appropriate
5. Motivational
6. Measurable

Resiliency

When adolescents suffer from low self-esteem, they may have difficulty in setting and attaining goals. They are afraid of failing. However, many not only survive in the face of adversity, but do well in life. Researchers in different countries discovered that some children and youths had developed specific skills, social competencies and attitudes that helped them to handle stress and chronic diseases. They also learned that the greater the number of protective factors (e.g. supportive family, educational standards) existing in their lives, the more likely they were to develop resiliency [O'Dougherty, 1983; Rutter, 1980; Werner, 1992].

Resiliency is the ability to adapt to changes and transitions, and/or deal with difficult problems and situations in a positive way. It is a quality that can be nurtured and developed in all children and adolescents, not just the ones growing up in adverse environments. Building resiliency is a positive approach to drug and violence prevention and any other behavior that puts a child, teen or young adult at risk. The focus is on strengthening the personal and environmental factors that contribute to the resiliency of young people. There are many ways in which clinicians can enhance protective factors for adolescents.

How to Build Resiliency

1. Build on the adolescent's cognitive, social, goal-oriented, physical, and civic competencies.
2. Promote a positive environment by setting high achievable standards for all youths.
3. Provide accurate, factual information from which patients can draw conclusions about the benefits and dangers of behaviors.
4. Encourage strong ties to the family and community.

Optimizing Self-Management Skills and Compliance via Health Education

Remember that giving only factual information to adolescents is less effective than an interactive health guidance process. However, busy clinicians rarely use this approach. As discussed in Chapter 1, providing *information* or *advice* alone is insufficient to promote behavioral *change* and *motivate* adolescents to comply with medical advice. Effective co-management of chronic disease requires an interactive approach, so that the adolescent and physician can share and listen to each other and express ideas about management issues. A joint plan of action is necessary for good management. The physician and adolescent must agree on the management plan in order to have a positive effect on clinical outcomes.

Techniques for Optimal Effectiveness of Management of Chronic Medical Conditions
1. Create agreements with the adolescent on the nature and extent of the chronic condition.
2. Determine the adolescent's attitude towards the condition, his or her level of knowledge regarding the condition, and motivation to co-manage the condition.
3. Reinforce healthy behaviors and health choices that improve the condition.
4. Determine with the adolescent a concrete, personalized course of management.
5. Encourage the adolescent to commit to this plan, and provide positive reinforcement when success is achieved.
6. Enlist family members to be supportive and collaborate with proper management when appropriate.
7. Arrange follow-up contacts on a regular basis.

Specific Issues: Asthma, Diabetes, Eating Disorders

Three chronic medical conditions — asthma, diabetes, and eating disorders — impact the quality of life of adolescents to a great extent, often altering their tasks of adolescent development.

Asthma

Asthma in adolescents is generally treated by intermittently-updated, standard protocols which have clinical evidence for the specific recommendations based on the most current efficacy research. The principles of asthma care can be gleaned from standard pediatric [Marks, 2010] and internal medicine textbooks, and guidelines may be found at Global Initiative for Asthma: www.ginasthma.com. This section will only give an overview with key recommendations and special considerations for adolescents.

> A 16-year-old male, Jon, was using his albuterol inhaler (without a spacer) about twice a week for episodes of wheezing, which were worse when he had colds, and sometimes occurred when he played sports. He had a night cough frequently, and had known allergies to house dust, which caused him to awake every morning with a stuffy nose. His doctor made suggestions for bedroom allergy control, some of which he did, including putting plastic casings on his bedding. Jon had a prescription for an inhaler of beclomethasone (ICS) to use twice a day on a regular basis, which he never obtained, preferring to use the albuterol inhaler

to control his cough and wheezing episodes. Finally, his physician would no longer refill his albuterol inhaler until he obtained the beclomethasone inhaler, and proved that he was using it with a spacer twice a day for prevention. Within 2 weeks, his wheezing episodes virtually stopped, and by adding a mild antihistamine at bedtime, his stuffy nose at night resolved. He was then able to limit his albuterol inhaler use (now with a spacer) to about once a month, mostly for exercise-induced wheezing.

Facilitating the use of preventive asthma medications and the evaluation of adequacy of asthma control are the keys to the treatment of asthmatic adolescents. There are several useful methods for evaluation of asthma control.

Rule of 2s:

Asthma is poorly controlled if there is
- 2 times a week daytime cough (not counting sick days).
- 2 times a month nighttime cough (not counting sick days).
- 2 times a year albuterol refills.
- 2 times a year unscheduled office visits.
- 2 times a year oral corticosteroids.

Past Month Asthma Control Test:

During the past 4 weeks
- How much time did your asthma keep you from getting as much done at work, school or at home? 1. All of the time; 2. Most of the time; 3. Some of the time; 4. A little of the time; 5. None of the time.
- How often have you had shortness of breath? 1. More than once a day; 2. Once a day; 3. 3–6 times a week; 4. Once or twice a week; 5. Rarely.
- How often did your asthma symptoms (wheezing, coughing, shortness of breath, chest tightness or pain) wake you up at night or earlier than usual in the morning? 1. 4 or more nights a week; 2. 2–3 nights a week; 3. Once a week; 4. Once or twice a month; 5. Rarely.
- How often have you used your rescue inhaler or nebulizer medication (such as albuterol)? 1. 3 or more times per day; 2. 1–2 times per day; 3. 2–3 times per week; 4. Once a week or less; 5. Not at all.
- How would you rate your asthma control? 1. Not controlled at all; 2. Poorly controlled; 3. Somewhat controlled; 4. Well controlled; 5. Completely controlled.

Add up the point values for each response to all five questions. If the total is less than 20, asthma may not be well controlled.

Quick Evaluation:
- Do you use albuterol for asthma symptoms more than 2 times a week, not counting use for exercise?
- Are you awakened from sleep by asthma symptoms (cough, wheeze, chest tightness, shortness of breath) more than two times a month?

If either is answered "Yes", it suggests poor control of asthma.

Review the Past Asthma History:
- Number of office visits for asthma the past 4 months, past 12 months.
- Number of ER visits for asthma in the past 4 months, past 12 months.
- Number of hospital admissions for asthma in the past 12 months.
- Last overnight hospital admission due to asthma was; 1. In the last 24 hours; 2. Less than 1 week ago; 3. Less than 1 month ago.

The diagnosis of a severity classification will determine which asthma treatment approach and medication is optimal and recommended. Four levels of asthma severity can be diagnosed: 1. Mild Intermittent, 2. Mild Persistent, 3. Moderate Persistent, and 4. Severe Persistent. Six questions can determine this diagnosis when the most severe level below is selected:

A. During the past 2 months, does the patient usually cough, wheeze or have trouble breathing during the day more than two times a week?
    If no → Mild Intermittent (go to B.)
    If yes, ask: Is it every day, all day long?
        If yes → Severe Persistent (stop)
        If no, ask: Is it once a day, every day?
            If no → Mild Persistent (go to B.)
            If yes → Moderate Persistent (go to B.)
B. During the past 2 months, does the patient usually cough, wheeze or have trouble breathing during the night more than two times a month?
    If no → Mild Intermittent (stop)
    If yes, ask: Is it three or more nights per week?
        If yes → Severe Persistent (stop)
        If no, ask: Is it more than one night per week?
            If no → Mild Persistent
            If yes → Moderate Persistent

Evidence-Based Treatment Approaches for Persistent Asthmatics
- Grade A evidence (++): Inhaled corticosteroids are strongly recommended as first line controller medications for persistent asthmatics.

- Grade B evidence (+): For children and youths who cannot take inhaled corticos-teroids (intolerant, decline, contraindicated), then leukotriene receptor antagonists (LTRA) (i.e. Singulair or nedocromil sodium) are alternative first line controller medications. In youths, adding a second agent such as a long-acting beta-agonist (LABA) (i.e. Serevent) is recommended. For exercise-induced asthma, short acting beta-agonist 5–15 min prior to exercise is recommended as initial therapy.
- Grade C evidence (+/−): For children and youths where inhaled corticosteroids alone do not give good control, adding LTRA is an option (works better for atopics).
- Grade D evidence (−): Long-acting beta-agonists (i.e. salmeterol) and cromolyn are not first line treatment for persistent asthma. Addition of cromolyn to inhaled corticosteroids is not recommended for uncontrolled patients.

Asthma Care Recommendations

Use an asthma action plan sheet (Fig. 4.1)! Use inhaled corticosteroids as first line treatment for persistent asthmatics. If additional treatment is needed, then add a long-acting beta-agonist (never give it by itself). Reevaluate every 1–6 months, and gradually reduce the dose of inhaled corticosteroid stepwise when asthma control is sustained for at least 3 months. Asthmatics should *never* smoke, since the long-term sequelae are horrible. Patient education, ongoing evaluation of compliance and avoidance of triggers (including smoking) are important for optimal management (Fig. 4.2).

Stepwise treatment approaches for persistent asthmatics

Step 1: Low-dose ICS (alternative: cromolyn, LTRA, nedocromil, or theophylline)
If good compliance and poor control:
Step 2: Low-dose ICS + LABA (= Advair100/50) or Medium-dose ICS (alternative: Low-dose ICS + either LTRA or theophylline or zileuton)

Diabetes

Diabetes mellitus (DM) in adolescents is generally treated by intermittently-updated, standard protocols which have clinical evidence for the specific recommendations based on the most current efficacy research. The principles of diabetes care can be gleaned from standard pediatric and internal medicine textbooks [Hofmann, Greydanus, 1997], and guidelines may be found at www.diabetesvoice.org and www.ada.org. This section will only give an overview with key recommendations and special considerations for adolescents.

Peak flow meter personal **BEST is:** _____

GREEN = GO ! Use your preventive medicine(s) daily, even if you are well. **If you don't use these every day, they will not work.**
This is where you should be every day. • Breathing is good • No coughing, wheezing, or shortness of breath • Can do activities or work **or** Peak Flow Number above _____ (Greater than 80% of BEST)   Daily **Preventive Medicines** are: _____ Before sports, use: _____
YELLOW = CAUTION ! Take your quick-relief medicines to keep from **getting worse. Keep taking your preventive medicine.**
You may have an asthma episode soon if you do not take proper action. • Cough or wheeze • Wake up at night with coughing, wheezing or shortness of breath • Increased breathing rate • First sign of a cold (if they often cause you to wheeze) • Tight chest **or** Peak Flow Number _____to_____ **Reliever Medicines** are: _____ Call your doctor if you don't return to your green zone.
RED = STOP ! Take rescue medicine now. If you are still is not better, **ask someone to take you to the hospital or clinic NOW.**
You should contact or see your doctor right away! • Medicine is not helping • Pulse is fast • Nose open wide when breathing • Hard to walk • Ribs or neck muscles show when breathing • It is hard to talk • Lips or fingernails turn gray or blue **or** Peak Flow Number below _____ (Less than 50% of BEST)   **Rescue Medicines** are: _____

Fig. 4.1   Asthma action plan.

Diagnosis of Type 1 Diabetes

The majority of DM type 1 is diagnosed in patients under 30 years old who are not obese. Common symptoms include thirst, urination, nocturia, and increased appetite, yet weight loss. Occasional symptoms include blurred vision, urinary tract infection,

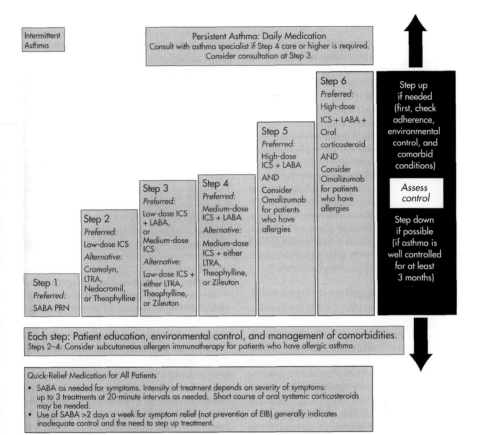

Fig. 4.2 Stepwise approach to therapy ages ≥ 12 years.

yeast infection, fatigue, acute abdominal pain, and flu-like symptoms. Urine ketones are usually positive, with or without diabetic ketoacidosis. The diagnosis is made with a random plasma glucose (RPG) of ≥ 200 mg/dL plus symptoms, or 8-hour fasting plasma glucose (FPG) of ≥ 126 mg/dL or oral glucose tolerance test (OGTT) 2-hour glucose value ≥ 200 mg/dL plus positive ketones. Hemoglobin A1C of 6.5 or above is also diagnostic. Prediabetes is diagnosed when Hgb A1c is 5.7–6.4. In the absence of acute metabolic decompensation, confirm it with a FPG within 24 hours. Diagnosis usually occurs under age 30, but type 1 diabetes can develop at any age. The presence of moderate to large serum ketones strongly suggests type 1 diabetes. See Fig. 4.3 for diagnostic considerations.

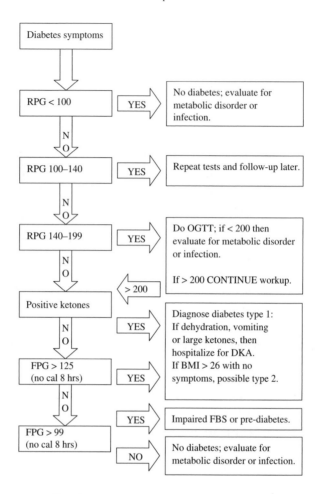

Fig. 4.3   Screening and diagnosis of type 1 diabetes.

A 75-gram Oral Glucose Tolerance Test is useful for diagnosing both type 1 and type 2 diabetes.
(Ingest 75 grams anhydrous glucose load dissolved in water; blood sugar 2 hours later)

Fasting	2 hours	=	Diagnosis
100–125	<140		Impaired fasting glucose
126–140	140–200		Impaired glucose tolerance
126–140	>200		Diabetes
>140	N/A		Diabetes

Initial Management of Diabetic Ketoacidosis (DKA)

Laboratory evaluation should include pH, electrolytes, glucose, urinalysis and urine ketones. Venous pH measurements have been found to accurately demonstrate the degree of acidosis of adult emergency department patients presenting with DKA, and should be used instead of arterial pH measurements. Urine ketone test is a better screening tool for DKA than the anion gap or serum bicarbonate.

Fluids: Assume about 15% dehydration. It is best to begin with a no bolus, or a maximum of 10 cc/kg bolus of normal saline or lactated ringer initially to treat clinical hemodynamic instability. A 5 cc/kg bolus can be repeated if hemodynamic instability persists. (Over-hydration has been associated with cerebral edema most often in children aged less than 5 years old.) There have been recommendations by many to begin with a 10-cc bolus and end with a 20-cc bolus in the absence of overt shock. (There are studies in children that demonstrate a significant mortality associated with more than 25 cc/kg within the first 4 hours of therapy.) The remainder of the fluid deficit is replaced using normal saline. It is recommended to begin with normal saline over the first 6 hours as the initial fluid in the infusate in order to minimize the free water intake. Maximum fluid intake by the patient for a 24-hour period should not exceed 4 liters per square meter to minimize the risk of cerebral edema.

Insulin recommendations are 0.1 unit per kilo per hour of insulin via IV drip. It is no longer recommended to give 0.1 unit per kilo bolus at the initial onset of therapy. Bicarbonate therapy is recommended only for patients who are in shock, respiratory depression, or with pH less than 7.0 with mental status changes.

Nutrition for DM-1 is based on body weight — use calculating tools (Exchange Book, Food Pyramid, etc.) to determine caloric needs, carbohydrates, and overall balanced nutrition. Adolescents newly diagnosed with diabetes should have a visit by an inpatient registered dietician while in hospital. This should include reinforcement of dietary regimens and to confirm an outpatient follow-up appointment in 1 month. Regular telephone follow-up with the dietician is helpful.

Outpatient and Home Management of Mild DKA

Management of mild ketosis in adolescents and young adults with diabetes can be attempted for a select group at home or in the outpatient setting. Candidates for this would-be patients with experienced families and a pH of > 7.3, a bicarbonate of > 15, able and willing to tolerate oral intake, normal mental status, less than 24 hours of symptoms of illness, previously good glucose control, and educated and comfortable in self-management of diabetes and the potential complications.

Patients should always check their ketones twice a day whenever they have an illness or whenever their capillary plasma blood glucose (PBG) is over 240. Most meters now provide readings adjusted to the "equivalent" of PBG. They must continue insulin since ketosis is due to the relative insulin deficiency. For mild ketosis, it is suggested that 10% of the total daily dose be given as human regular (R) or rapid-acting (RA) insulin. For moderate or large ketones, it is suggested that 15–20% of the total daily insulin dose be given as R or RA insulin. Patients should recheck the urine ketones in 3 hours and repeat the same procedures if ketones are still present. Continue to repeat this process every 3 hours until the ketones are gone. It is important to keep the PBG > 200 or whole blood glucose (WBG) > 180 prior to any Regular insulin injections. It is also important to ensure that the patient is well educated on DM management, is not severely ill, and is comfortable doing this regimen. Should the patient be unable to tolerate oral fluids, become more ketotic or more ill while using this regimen, he or she should be seen by a physician or go to the emergency room for further evaluation.

Guidelines for Ongoing Care

A multidisciplinary adolescent diabetes management team should include team members consisting of a physician, diabetes nurse clinician, dietitian, behavioral health specialist and a certified diabetes educator (CDE). The implementation of recommended practice guidelines will optimize patient care.

Roles and Responsibilities
- Family: Provision of physical, emotional, medical, educational needs.
- Patient: Attend school or work, family and personal responsibilities, diabetes self-management.
- Health provider: Medical care, advice and education, appointments, support, social services support when needed, and referral to endocrinology when appropriate.

Treatment options involve insulin dosed intermittently (or through a pump) and synchronized with both a food plan and exercise program. Type 1 patients require insulin therapy and should not be treated with an oral agent. More than 50% of self-monitored blood glucose (SMBG) values should be within target range. The patient should use a meter with memory and also keep a log book. Monitoring is done a minimum of four times per day (before every meal and before a bedtime snack). Periodically check 2 hours after the start of meals, and sometimes at 3 a.m. as needed for morning hyperglycemia or nocturnal hypoglycemia.

SMBG Targets for DM Type 1
- Age 13–19 years: PBG 90–130 mg/dl at pre-meal, and 90–150 mg/dl at bedtime.
- Age ≥ 20 years: PBG 70–130 mg/dl at pre-meal, and < 200 mg/dl at 1–2 hours post prandial.
- With no severe (assisted) or nocturnal hypoglycemia.

Adjust pre-meal target upwards if there is hypoglycemia unawareness or repeated severe hypoglycemia episodes. The patient should always check urine ketones if PBG is over 240 on two consecutive occasions, or if any illness or infection is present. Most meters read the "equivalent" of PBG. Total glycosylated hemoglobin (HgbA1c) can be used to verify SMBG data or if no SMBG data available. If possible, obtain it prior to a clinic visit to assist in clinical decision making. If HgbA1c does not correlate with SMBG, check meter accuracy, assess patient SMBG skills, monitor WBG more frequently, and/or refer for diabetes education.

Targets for Hemoglobin A_{1C}

- Age 6–12 years: < 8.0.
- Age 13–19 years: < 7.5.
- Age ≥ 20 years: Target < 7.0.
- Frequency 3–4 times per year [ADA Guidelines].

Monthly office visits are necessary during insulin adjustment phases, and weekly phone contact may be necessary. Suggestions for pattern adjustments are:

- Determine which insulin is responsible for pattern.
- Adjust only one dose at a time.
- Correct hypoglycemia first.
- If total dose >1.5 Unit/kg, consider over-insulinization.
- If hyperglycemia occurs throughout the day, correct highest SMBG first.
- If all within 50 mg/dL of target, correct the AM first.

Insulin Adjustments of R (Regular) or RA (Rapid-Acting) Insulin:

- Adjust at times of R or RA insulin injections.
- May be added or subtracted on basis of PBG, food, or exercise.
- Use with caution at bedtime; 3 AM PBG is used to determine the bedtime dose.

PBG as pre-meal (meter equivalent)

	Adjust R or RA
< 70	down 1 Unit
70–150	no change
150–200	up 1 Unit
201–250	up 2 Units
250–300	up 3 Units
301–350	up 4 Units
> 350	up 5 Units
	(may need more if overweight or obese)

Other insulin management adjustments include: Evaluate nocturnal hypoglycemia by checking 3 a.m. SMBG; consider adjusting bedtime snack. Other possible adjustments to consider: adding or adjusting mid-morning snack; adding or adjusting afternoon snack; adding exercise; evaluate if previous exercise is causing hypoglycemia. Morning long-acting insulin (LA) is basal and usually does not require adjusting. If PM SMBG is greater than target due to a long interval between midday and evening meals, consider increasing LA by 1–2 units. Human NPH insulin (N) may be needed at times to cover snacks or different eating patterns, rather than using RA insulin for covering a snack immediately. Whenever there is erratic SMBG control or weight gain, and total insulin dose is over 1.0–1.5 Unit/kg, this suggests possible over-insulinization. Consider decreasing total daily dose to 1.0 Unit/kg and redistributing doses: AM = 25% N and 25% R; Lunch = 10% R; Dinner = 25% R or mix; Bedtime = 15% R or mix.

Adolescents who are candidates for an insulin pump must have sufficient knowledge and self-management skills, as well as willingness to monitor PBG 4–7 times a day. They should already have good diabetes control, problem-solving ability, motivation, understanding and successful use of carbohydrate counting, good nutrition, and must have excellent hypoglycemia recognition. Pump insulin is usually 40% basal, and 60% bolus, which is adjusted based on food distribution. A pump is usually initiated with the assistance of an endocrinologist and a pump trainer or certified diabetes educator.

Every 3–4 months, diabetic adolescents should be reevaluated regarding: hypoglycemia, medications, weight, height or BMI, food plan and exercise, BP, SMBG data (download meter), HgbA1c, foot check, diabetes/nutrition continuing education, smoking cessation, as well as contraceptive (or pre-pregnancy) planning. A dietician should be seen at least every 6–12 months. An annual comprehensive evaluation should be done, which includes history and physical, fasting lipid profile, dilated eye examination, dental examination, neurologic assessment, and a complete foot examination. Blood pressure target is: <130/80. Lipid targets are: LDL <130, HDL $\geq$ 50 mg/dL, triglyceride <150 mg/dL. An annual urine spot microalbumin/creatinine ratio is also performed and should be less than 30. If it is greater than 30, then repeat it three times within a 6-month period. If 2 out of 3 tests are in the range 30–300, then obtain a 24-hour urine creatinine, follow BP, and begin treatment with Lisinopril/ACE inhibitors. If any results are greater than 300, then obtain a 24-hour urine protein/creatinine ratio, and refer for further evaluation for other medical causes, as well as treatment.

Diagnosis of Type 2 Diabetes

Type 2 diabetes has become nearly epidemic in many countries where obesity is prevalent, particularly among populations of people who are sedentary and eating Western diets.

Carrie is a 16-year-old female with presumed DM type 2 who is overweight. In August, her height was at the 75th percentile (166 cm) and her weight (101 kg) was well above 95th percentile, with a BMI of 36. She had a fasting glucose of 137 (normal range 70–99 mg/dl), and her TSH was 2.07 (normal: 0.35–5.50 uIU/ml). Her lipid panel revealed: cholesterol 243 (normal: < 176 mg/dl), triglyceride 256 (normal: < 126 mg/dl), HDL 35 (normal: > 59 mg/dl), and LDL 157 (normal: 10–110 mg/dl). She was referred to the dietician for intensive dietary education, and told to return in 1 month. She returned in 2 months, in October, and at that time her weight was unchanged, her fasting glucose was 139, her HgbA1c was 6.5, and she was given a glucometer with instructions to use it four times a day and keep records of her sugars to bring back in 2 weeks at a return visit. She was scheduled for an interim follow-up with the dietician. She returned 6 months later in April, and had a fasting glucose of 111, a HgbA1c % of 6.2, and her lipid panel revealed: cholesterol 267, triglyceride 241, HDL 37, LDL 182. She was prescribed metformin, which caused nausea and was not tolerated. She did not return to the office until she needed a physical for school 3 months later, and her weight was 99 kg. Her parents were counseled in depth about expectations for her continued care, and she was assigned to a care management team for strict follow-up according to guidelines.

Type 2 Diabetes Risk Factors

- Overweight (defined as BMI > 85th percentile for age and sex, weight for height > 85th percentile, or weight > 120% of ideal weight for height).
- Family history of type 2 diabetes in first or second degree relative.
- Racial/ethnic group: Asian, Pacific Islander, Hispanic, African, Native American.
- Signs of insulin resistance: acanthosis nigricans, hypertension, dyslipidemia, polycystic ovary syndrome.

See Fig. 4.4 for diagnostic considerations. If the adolescent is obese, or if type 1 diabetes is suspected, consider measuring insulin level by C-peptide, which may be low/normal in type 1 diabetes and high/normal in type 2 diabetes.

Possible treatment activities for type 2 diabetes include fitness testing, weight programs, portion control, and carbohydrate counting. Initiate and continue with diabetes self management education and training, as well as medical nutrition therapy throughout all stages of treatment. Surveillance for CVD, renal, retinal, neurological, and foot disease are also important for type 2. In type 2 diabetes, when FPG is greater than 300 at diagnosis or urine ketones with FPG more than 200, then insulin should be considered for management. Hospitalization should be considered

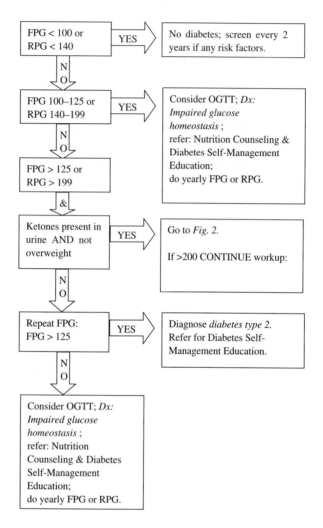

Fig. 4.4   Screening and diagnosis of type 2 diabetes.

if ketones are present or if the patient is unable to implement initial treatments. Metformin side effects are usually dose-related and self-limited, and commonly include diarrhea, nausea, and abdominal discomfort, and occasionally a metallic taste. Precautions and contraindications for metformin include pregnancy and lactation, and when there exists a risk of lactic acidosis in patients with renal disease (plasma creatinine $>1.4\,mg/dl$), liver dysfunction, alcohol abuse, binge drinking, acute or chronic metabolic acidosis, acute cardiovascular or pulmonary disease, and also with

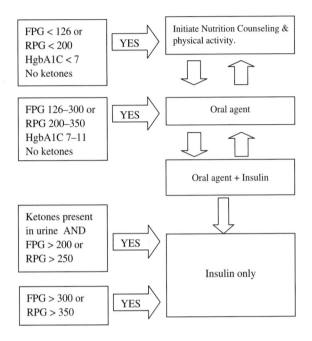

Fig. 4.5   Management of type 2 diabetes.

intravenous radiographic contrast agents (stop at time of procedure, resume 2 days after, and once renal function is found to be normal). See Fig. 4.5 for treatment considerations.

SMBG testing should be done 1–4 times a day, and sometimes 2 hours after the start of a meal. When using insulin, testing should be done four times a day. HgbA1c should be kept under 7.0. There should be no severe (assisted) or nocturnal hypoglycemia, and more than 50% of PBG readings are expected within these target ranges: before meals should be 90–130; 2 hours after start of meal should be less than 200; and bedtime in the range 90–150.

Eating disorders are somewhat common in the adolescent diabetic population, and purposeful omission of insulin (or under-dosing) is considered a form of eating disorder, commonly found among teen girls who are trying to lose weight (or remain thin), and do so by remaining in borderline DKA.

Eating Disorders

Exercise is king, nutrition is queen — put them together and you've got a kingdom.

—Jack LaLanne

Obesity and Overweight

Healthy eating in adolescence is important for growth and development and prevents health problems such as obesity, dental caries, and iron deficiency anemia. Probably a quarter of adolescents do not eat breakfast. Food insufficiency is associated with behavioral problems and poor academic functioning. Based on social and economic conditions in many areas around the world, certain groups of adolescents are significantly undernourished. Few adolescents worldwide eat fruits and vegetables five times daily. A healthy diet is associated with lowered risk for many diseases, including three leading causes of death: cancer, heart disease, and stroke. In many westernized countries, many adolescents exceed dietary allowances for total fat and saturated fat intake. Early signs of atherosclerosis, the major cause of heart disease, begin in adolescence (or earlier), and it is related to high cholesterol levels, often caused by poor dietary habits. Parental levels of obesity and their food preferences also affect children's preferences.

In many parts of the world, the prevalence of overweight children aged 6–11 years more than doubled from 1980 to 2000, and overweight adolescents aged 12–19 more than tripled, increasing from 5% to 18%. This is likely due to the progressive sedentary lifestyle brought on partly by television and computer screens. American adolescents spend more time watching television than in any other activity except sleeping. Television also displaces time spent on other calorie-using activities. There is a strong association between television and computer screen viewing time and obesity. In fact, a 2% increase in the prevalence of obesity has been documented for each extra hour of daily television viewing by those 12–17 years of age. Having a television set in the bedroom is a strong predictor of being overweight.

Fast food restaurants have completely changed the way adolescents eat worldwide and contribute significantly to the problem of obesity. In the year 2000, Americans spent $110 billion on fast food — more than on higher education, computers, or cars. Many adolescents now get over 10% of their total energy intake from fast foods, compared with 2% in the late 1970s. From 1970 to 1995, the number of fast food restaurants worldwide more than doubled, providing foods with much more fat and sugar. For the first 10 years of the 21st century, as of 2010, approximately 5% of adolescents are obese, and as many as 25% are overweight. Type 2 diabetes, high blood pressure, high cholesterol and asthma have become increasingly prevalent among adolescents as rates of overweight and obesity rise. It has been said that, due to obesity, this generation of adolescents may not outlive their parents.

Adolescence appears to be a crucial period when overweight and obesity can occur. In males, abdominal fat is deposited; in females, the percentage of body fat increases.

Puberty is also a time of relative insulin resistance. In addition, early menarche carries a two-fold increased risk of being overweight. Overweight and obese teenagers have an 80% likelihood of becoming overweight and obese adults. Adolescents are more physically active than adults, but participation in physical activity declines with age in adolescence. In many westernized countries, many adolescents do not engage in moderate or vigorous physical activity at least 3 days a week. Physical activity directly reduces the risk of hypertension and diabetes mellitus, as well as later coronary heart disease and colon cancer. Regular physical activity in adolescence improves strength and endurance, builds strong bones and muscles, controls weight, reduces emotional anxiety and depression, increases self-esteem, and may improve blood pressure and cholesterol levels. Health-related fitness includes cardio-respiratory endurance, muscular strength and endurance, flexibility, and body composition; skill-related fitness includes reaction time, speed, balance, agility, power, and coordination.

The clinician should determine the patient's BMI using a BMI chart to identify at-risk adolescents; weight and height measurements are converted to body mass index (BMI). $BMI = Weight (kg)/Height (m^2)$. Overweight is defined as a BMI of 25–30 (85–95th percentile), and obese is a BMI over the 95th percentile (>30). Overweight and obesity are disturbances in basic energy balance: what goes in exceeds what is used. Weight gain is caused by a very small imbalance occurring over a long period of time. Obesity itself is considered a chronic disease which, like others, impairs the body's normal functioning, decreases life expectancy, can cause death and, like other diseases, can be inherited. Only about 2% of obesity is associated with any medical cause or identifiable endocrine abnormality.

Many obese adolescents are also tall for their age. Obese patients who are short for their age are more likely to have an endocrine or genetic syndrome causing obesity. Height, weight and BMI should be plotted for age at every visit. Blood pressure should be measured using an appropriately sized cuff. The physical examination should include a fundoscopic examination to evaluate for blurring of optic discs, which may indicate pseudotumor cerebri. The thyroid must be examined for signs of enlargement. Sexual maturity rating should be done on every patient to evaluate pubertal stage. The skin should be examined for signs of acanthosis nigricans (thick, pigmented skin over the neck and sometimes upper chest).

Obese females often begin puberty earlier than non-obese peers, whereas most endocrine causes of obesity cause poor height growth. Adolescents with Cushing's disease, hypothyroidism, or growth hormone deficiency present with short stature and obesity. Irregular menses are associated to thyroid dysfunction; females with regular menses rarely have a thyroid disorder. Avoid unnecessary testing — obese females at

Tanner 4 or 5, at or over the 75th percentile for height with regular menses do not need thyroid function testing such as a screening TSH. Endocrine laboratory screening for overweight patients is rarely needed, but screening of lipid levels are recommended by age 21. Fasting glucose screening for type 2 diabetes is recommended. About a third of obese children have symptoms of sleep apnea and sometimes Pickwickian syndrome.

"Metabolic syndrome" presents with clinical features of insulin resistance: 1. Acanthosis nigricans; 2. Accelerated or slowed linear growth; or 3. Polycycstic ovarian disease (PCOS). Although there are no specific diagnostic criteria for the syndrome in adolescents, it is typically diagnosed when patients have three or more of the following criteria:

- BMI > 95% for age and sex,
- BP > 95% for age and sex,
- Triglycerides > 95% for age and sex,
- HDL < 5% for age and sex, and
- Impaired fasting glucose > 100 mg/dl or impaired glucose tolerance > 140 mg/dl.

Clinicians should counsel adolescents to increase physical activity and decrease sedentary activity. Simply cutting TV and computer time in half will often result in a significant weight loss. Every adolescent should habitually engage in three or more sessions per week of activities that last at least 20 minutes with moderate to vigorous levels of exertion. Preventively, normal children in westernized countries should switch to skim or 1% milk at 2 years of age. Adolescents often drink sodas, and increased consumption of soft drinks and fruit juices is clearly associated to weight gain and a significant risk of type 2 diabetes in young women [Schulze *et al.*, 2004]. A can of soda contains 150 calories, and if consumed daily, this is equivalent to 15 pounds of weight gain a year. Adolescents should drink diet sodas rather than regular sugared soda.

Changing one's lifestyle is more effective in long-term weight management than "going on a diet." However, learning the caloric content of foods eaten in a typical day is often an eye opener, particularly if one scrutinizes the serving sizes (servings per container) on typical food labels. As of this writing, food labels are misleading since most people who eat the contents of a container of food usually think they are eating one serving with the listed caloric and fat content, but it is necessary to multiply these by the number of servings in the container! A useful lifestyle recommendation can be: "If you believe you are hungry, you may actually be thirsty. Drink a glass of water and wait 20 minutes. If you are still hungry, eat fruit and vegetables." Successful treatments have five component requirements:

1. Decreases in caloric intake.
2. Increased physical activity.

3. Behavior modification and psychological support.
4. Family involvement and collaboration.
5. Regular clinical contacts.

Management of Overweight Patients

- Make the diagnosis of overweight or obese.
- Assess with directed history and physical.
- Exclude associated medical problems with laboratory studies.
- Determine adolescent's readiness for change (Prochaska).
- Counsel diet, activity, follow-up plans.
- Refer to dietician and other effective programs when available.
- Schedule ongoing clinical contacts and support.

Useful Weight Loss Measures

- Set a goal to lose 2 pounds a month.
- Keep a diary (for 1 week) of all food intake and activity (used for calorie count by dietician).
- Adjust food purchases — limit high-calorie foods both outside and in the home.
- Assess and address obstacles.
- Arrange family and peer support for weight loss.
- Reward successes.

Weight management involves the entire family. One goal is to adjust the way the entire family shops, eats, and exercises. Overweight or obesity is not just the adolescent's problem; it is the family's problem. Additionally, school and community programs that promote regular physical activity among adolescents are highly cost-effective ways to reduce the public health burden of chronic diseases associated with sedentary lifestyles. Programs that provide students with the knowledge, attitudes, motor skills, behavioral skills, and confidence to participate in physical activity may establish active lifestyles among adolescents that continue into and throughout their adult lives.

Anorexia and Bulimia

"Under-eating" disorders may be the third most common chronic condition in adolescents (after obesity and asthma), and they are notoriously challenging to treat. Bulimia nervosa is more common than anorexia nervosa, which can occur in up to 5% of adolescent females. Over 90% of all eating disorders occur in adolescent females. Cultural, social, and environmental factors, as well as psychological factors in both the adolescent and the family, contribute to the development of eating disorders [Pathy, 2008].

Anorexia nervosa is the unwillingness to keep body weight at or above the minimal normal weight for age. There is a fear of gaining weight or being fat, even though the patient is clinically underweight. It is a psychological disturbance of perception and experience of body weight or shape with denial of the magnitude of the problem. Females have amenorrhea for at least three consecutive menstrual cycles. The onset of menses may be delayed if disordered eating begins before menarche. The "restricting type" includes persistent and severe caloric restriction, sometimes with compulsive exercise. There is no binge-eating or purging. A strong desire to be thin leads to progressive weight loss. The "binge eating or purging type" involves restriction as well as intermittent bulimic episodes with self-induced vomiting or use of laxatives, diuretics, or enemas. The anorectic adolescent may be malnourished and have signs and symptoms including constipation, cold intolerance, hair loss, dizziness, light-headedness, as well as emotional symptoms such as irritability or depression. An appearance of depression is usually caused by starvation, however. Presenting complaints may include primary or secondary amenorrhea, abdominal pain, syncope, weight loss, or failure to gain weight as expected, but usually the adolescent has no complaint when the parents bring in their teen.

The bulimia nervosa patient may have any weight or body type, and there are often no signs or symptoms. There may be binge-eating immediately followed by some action to eliminate the ingested food. Purging (self-induced vomiting, or laxative, emetic, enema or diuretic use) is done by most patients with bulimia nervosa. The major criteria of bulimia nervosa is not the purging, but the recurrent episodes of binge-eating with a feeling that the patient cannot stop eating or control how much is eaten. The non-purging bulimic usually fasts or exercises to maintain or lose weight, or does other inappropriate compensatory behaviors, at least twice a week. Most female adolescents with bulimia have oligomenorrhea (menstrual irregularity) but not complete amenorrhea.

On physical examination, anorexic adolescents may show weight and body mass index below ideal body weight for height, hypothermia, bradycardia, or orthostasis. Hypotension occurs in severe cases. There may be a cardiac murmur (1 in 3 females have mitral valve prolapse), or hair loss, dry skin, or lanugo with peripheral edema or acrocyanosis. Signs of purging include eroded tooth enamel, parotid enlargement, or scars on the knuckles (Russell's sign) from using fingers to induce emesis. However, bulimics usually are normal weight or overweight. There may be cardiac arrhythmias (from electrolyte imbalance).

The diagnosis of eating disorders is made clinically, and laboratory tests only help to assess medical complications or identify other possible causes of weight loss such as diabetes or hyperthyroidism. Initial screening tests should include a complete blood count (malnutrition can show cytopenias), electrolytes (pH, sodium and potassium may be abnormal with abnormal water intake, vomiting, laxative or diuretic use), and check for abnormal urine specific gravity in anorexics who sometimes drink extra water before an office visit to add body weight. Additional tests may include: cholesterol (high in starvation), liver function tests (fatty liver), thyroid function tests (possibly low), and a sedimentation rate to rule out possible inflammatory bowel disease. Adolescents with amenorrhea for more than 6 months should have a scan for bone density to evaluate risk of osteopenia or osteoporosis. In the presence of significant bradycardia or purging, a prolonged QT interval from hypokalemia may be seen on electrocardiogram. Rarely, hormone tests in females with amenorrhea are indicated, but they may include luteinizing hormone, follicle-stimulating hormone, prolactin, and estradiol.

The differential diagnosis includes:
- Psychiatric: obsessive-compulsive disorder (OCD) or depression;
- Gastrointestinal: inflammatory bowel disease, malabsorption or celiac disease;
- Endocrine: diabetes, thyroid condition, Addison disease, hypopituitarism;
- Brain tumor, another chronic disease, or chronic infection such as human immunodeficiency virus (HIV).

Clinicians should identify variations of eating disorders that do not meet the full criteria for either anorexia or bulimia nervosa but still deserve medical and psychiatric attention. Growth stunting, failure to attain peak bone mineral mass, and structural brain changes are potentially irreversible complications of eating disorders in adolescents and provide the rationale for early diagnosis and aggressive treatment, especially in pre- and peripubertal children.

The optimal treatment of eating disorders requires a multidisciplinary team approach. Medical care, dietician services and mental health treatment must be coordinated. The key to recovery is nutrition, but antidepressant medications, especially selective serotonin reuptake inhibitors (SSRIs such as fluoxetine) are often helpful, and can also prevent relapse in recovering adolescents with anorexia. They are useful to treat the OCD symptoms and have an antibulimic effect that decreases binging and purging. Bupropion and tricyclic antidepressants should not be used. Though eating disorders are usually treated in outpatient centers, some severely malnourished adolescents will require inpatient hospitalization for enteral or parenteral nutrition. The mortality averages about 5%, resulting from suicide, cardiac dysfunction or electrolyte imbalance. Electrolyte monitoring in patients with bulimia is essential, as the risk is present for sudden cardiac death due to hypokalemia. About half of adolescents with anorexia nervosa recover completely, a third partly recover, and a fifth have little improvement.

Outpatient Eating Disorder Treatment

- Provide *education* on nutrition (healthy diet with adequate calories) and on appropriate exercise.
- Maximize *family support* and understanding using counseling and education, while countering co-dependency.
- Begin a rigorous *eating disorder protocol* with behavioral techniques to normalize eating patterns, eliminate purging behavior, lessen unhealthy eating behaviors and reward weight gain.
- Schedule *psychotherapy* (CBT) to change attitudes about eating and body image and to treat associated mood disorders.

The Dying Adolescent

Some adolescents die from the effects of chronic illnesses. It is challenging to provide appropriate terminal care for them because of developmental, social, and legal issues. Life-threatening illness affects the otherwise normal physical and psychological developmental changes for this age group (independence, peer interactions, self-image, etc.). Emotional and psychological regression is common during illness. Legally, few terminally-ill adolescents who have not yet reached adulthood can make medical decisions such as discontinuing medical interventions. It is therefore very important to facilitate early, optimal decision-making and communication between the dying adolescent, his or her family, and his or her medical team, so that the adolescent's true preferences are respected while maintaining self-determination. Progressive, graduated involvement in medical decisions by an adolescent becomes developmentally appropriate for matters such as choosing between cancer therapies, or discontinuing treatments after a number of relapses.

The clinician should strongly encourage truthfulness in disclosing the original diagnosis to an adolescent, which can help avoid the situation of a parent opposing disclosure of the terminal illness to the adolescent later. Moral arguments for truthfulness suggest that the clinician should inform parents that he or she will not lie to an adolescent if directly asked about issues concerning death. Parental reluctance usually represents a desire to protect their child and the inability to accept death; the truth will eventually reduce anxiety and increase trust by the adolescent. With any diagnosis or set of treatment options, it is ethically responsible to involve the adolescent in communication and decision options as much as is developmentally appropriate. All terminally-ill adolescents should be allowed to make palliative care decisions with maximal autonomy.

Suggested Readings and Bibliography

American Academy of Pediatrics. (2004). Preventing childhood obesity: a national conference focusing on pregnancy, infancy, and early childhood obesity. *Pediatrics,* 114, Suppl, p. i.

American Academy of Pediatrics. (2006). Eating disorders. *Pediatr Rev*, 27, pp. 5–15.

American Academy of Pediatrics Committee on Adolescence. (2003). Identifying and treating eating disorders. *Pediatrics*, 111, pp. 204–211.

American Academy of Pediatrics. Committee on Bioethics. (1994). Guidelines for forgoing life-sustaining medical treatment. *Pediatrics*, 93, pp. 532–536.

American Psychiatric Association. (1994). *Diagnostic and Statistical Manual of Mental Disorders*. 4th Edn. (American Psychiatric Association, Washington).

Bar-Or O, Baranowski T. (1994). Physical activity, adiposity, and obesity among adolescents. *Pediatr Exercise Sci*, 6, pp. 348–360.

Bean R. (1992). *The Four Conditions of Self-Esteem: A New Approach for Elementary and Middle Schools*. (ETR Associates, USA).

Benett PH, Haffner S, Kasiske BL, *et al.* (1995). Screening and management of microalbuminuria in patients with diabetes mellitus: recommendations to the Scientific Advisory Board of the National Kidney Foundation from an ad hoc committee of the Council on Diabetes Mellitus of the National Kidney Foundation. *Am J Kidney Dis*, 25, pp. 107–112.

Bhogal S, Zemek R, Ducharme FM. (2006). Written action plans for asthma in children. *Cochrane Database Syst Rev*, 3, CD005306.

Blum RW. (1987). Compliance in the adolescent with chronic illness. *Semin Adolesc Med*, 3, pp. 157–162.

Bowers WA. (2001). Basic principles for applying cognitive-behavioral therapy to anorexia nervosa. *Psychiatr Clin N Am*, 24, pp. 293–303.

Brandenburg MA, Dire DJ. (1998). Comparison of arterial and venous blood gas values in the initial emergency department evaluation of patients with diabetic ketoacidosis. *Ann Emerg Med*, 31, pp. 459–465.

Chase. (2006). *Understanding Diabetes: A handbook for people who are living with diabetes*. (Children's Diabetes Foundation at Denver, Denver).

Cooley WC. (2004). Redefining primary pediatric care for children with special health care needs: the primary care medical home. *Curr Opin Pediatr*, 16, pp. 689–692.

Daniels SR, Khoury PR, Morrison JA. (1997). The utility of body mass index as a measure of body fatness in children and adolescents: differences by race and gender. *Pediatrics*, 109, pp. 1028–1035.

Freyer D. (2004). Care of the dying adolescent: special considerations. *Pediatrics*, 113, pp. 381–388.

Haynes RB, Yao X, Degani A, *et al.* (2005). Interventions to enhance medication adherence. *Cochrane Database Syst Rev*, 4, CD000011.

Hein HO, Suadicani P, Gyntelberg F. (1992). Physical fitness or physical activity as a predictor of ischaemic heart disease? A 17-year follow-up in the Copenhagen Male Study. *J Intern Med*, 232, pp. 471–479.

Helmrich SP, Ragland DR, Leung RW, Paffenbarger RS Jr. (1991). Physical activity and reduced occurrence of non-insulin-dependent diabetes mellitus. *N Engl J Med*, 325, pp. 147–152.

Hofmann AD, Greydanus DE (eds). (1997). *Adolescent Medicine*. 3rd Edn. (McGraw-Hill/Appleton & Lange, USA). ISBN-10: 0838500676; ISBN-13: 978-0838500675.

International Diabetes Center. (1995). *Staged Diabetes Management: Decision Paths*. (Park Nicollet Medical Foundation, Minneapolis).

Kaufman FR. (1997). Diabetes mellitus. *Pediatr Rev*, 18, pp. 383–392.

Kaye WH, Nagata T, Weltzin TE, *et al.* (2001). Double-blind placebo-controlled administration of fluoxetine in restricting- and restricting-purging-type anorexia nervosa. *Biol Psychiatry*, 49, pp. 644–652.

Kitabchi AE, Wall BM. (1995). Diabetic ketoacidosis. *Med Clin North Am*, 79, pp. 9–37.

La Greca AM. (1998). It's "all in the family": responsibility for diabetes care. *J Pediatr Endocrinol Metab*, 11, Suppl 2, pp. 379–385.

La Greca AM, Bearman KJ. (2001). Commentary: if "an apple a day keeps the doctor away," why is adherence so darn hard? *J Pediatr Psychol*, 26, pp. 279–282.

Marks J. (2010). Pulmonology. In: Greydanus D, Patel D, Reddy V, Feinberg A, Omar H (eds), *Handbook of Clinical Pediatrics: An Update for the Ambulatory Pediatrician*, pp. 276–288. (World Scientific Publishing, Singapore).

National Heart, Lung, and Blood Institute; United States Department of Health and Human Services. (2007). Expert panel report 3: guidelines for the diagnosis and management of asthma: full report 2007 National Asthma Education and Prevention Program. NIH publication 08-4051. Available at: http://www.nhlbi.nih.gov/guidelines/asthma/

O'Dougherty M, Wright FS, Garmezy N, *et al.* (1983). Later competence and adaptation in infants who survive severe heart defects. *Child Dev*, 54, pp. 1129–1142.

Pathy P. (2008). Eating disorders. In: Fung D, Yiming C (eds), *A Primer of Child and Adolescent Psychiatry*, pp. 137–154. (World Scientific Publishing, Singapore).

Powell KE, Kreuter MW, Stephens T, Marti B, Heinemann L. (1991). The dimensions of health promotion applied to physical activity. *J Public Health Policy*, 12, pp. 492–509.

Robinson TN. (1999). Reducing children's television viewing to prevent obesity: a randomized controlled trial. *JAMA*, 282, pp. 1561–1567.

Roter DL, Hall JA, Merisca R, *et al.* (1998). Effectiveness of interventions to improve patient compliance: a meta-analysis. *Med Care*, 36, pp. 1138–1161.

Rutter M. (1980). School influences on children's behavior and development: the 1979 Kenneth Blackfan Lecture, Children's Hospital Medical Center, Boston. *Pediatrics*, 65, pp. 208–220.

Schnieder B. (2005). Obesity in children and adolescents. *Pediatr Rev*, 26, pp. 155–161.

Schulze MB, Manson JE, Ludwig DS, *et al.* (2004). Sugar-sweetened beverages, weight gain, and incidence of type 2 diabetes in young and middle-aged women. *JAMA*, 292, pp. 927–934.

Schwab TM, Hendey GW, Soliz TC. (1999). Screening for ketonemia in patients with diabetes. *Ann Emerg Med*, 34, pp. 342–346.

Steffes MW. (1997). Diabetic nephropathy: incidence, prevalence, and treatment. *Diabetes Care*, 20, pp. 1059–1060.

Trent M. (2002). Adolescent obesity: identifying a new risk of at-risk youth. *Pediatr Ann*, 31, pp. 559–564.

Vermeire E, Hearnshaw H, Van Royen P, Denekens J. (2001). Patient adherence to treatment: three decades of research. A comprehensive review. *J Clin Pharm Ther*, 26, pp. 331–342.

Werner EE. (1992). The children of Kauai: resiliency and recovery in adolescence and adulthood. *J Adolesc Health*, 13, pp. 262–268.

Wilson K, Klein J, Sesselberg T, *et al.* (2006). Use of complementary medicine and dietary supplements among US adolescents. *J Adolesc Health*, 38, pp. 385–394.

Suggested Websites

Global Initiative for Asthma: http://www.ginasthma.com

Principles of diabetes care: http://www.diabetesvoice.org

Just for Teens (American Diabetes Association): This page from the ADA provides diabetic teens with information about how to work with their health care team, effective communications, self-esteem, assertiveness, confidentiality, and telling friends about their disease. http://www.diabetes.org/for-parents-and-kids/for-teens.jsp

Chapter 5

Fatigue and Psychosomatic Illnesses

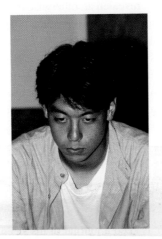

Overview

Fatigue is a common problem for adolescents, and it can be recurrent, persistent, prolonged or chronic. The feeling of sleepiness, from not having had enough sleep, is similar to weakness or tiredness. Fatigue can also be one of the many diffuse symptoms of stress-related problems, and that is why it is included in this chapter on psychosomatic illnesses.

Teenagers frequently worry about their bodies and their health. At least 10% of teenagers report either frequent headaches, chest pain, nausea, or fatigue. In a survey of 1500 middle school students, 25% reported headaches, 15% reported abdominal pains regularly, and 10% had other psychosomatic illnesses. However, clinicians often fail to identify psychosocial problems — 80% were not detected in some studies. Clinicians may under-report such problems because of concerns about insurance reimbursement or personal stigmatization.

Fatigue

There are a variety of fatigue states: Weakness is when muscles cannot do their usual work. Easy fatigability is tiring rapidly without much exertion. Fatigue itself is feeling tired as if not having had enough sleep.

A 20-year-old male presented to the clinic with 2 months of feeling "tired most of the time." He felt he had little energy, and complained of wanting to sleep when studying. The history revealed an otherwise healthy male with only a past knee injury. He said that he could not sleep well at night, which is why he stayed up until about 2 a.m. most nights and felt tired in the mornings. Further history revealed that many nights he was playing computer games online or watching television, since he could not fall asleep later. He denied any drug use or evening caffeine beverages, but routinely needed a 2-hour nap after dinner. He would arise at 7 a.m. three mornings a week to attend classes at junior college, and worked 4 days a week for 7 hours on the other days. The symptoms began 2 months ago when he had a severe flu, and he never felt totally recuperated, although he continued going to school and returned to his job after a few days. Psychosocial screening revealed no specific stressors or signs of depression. His complete physical examination was totally normal. He was advised to limit naps to 1 hour in the afternoon, to do no stimulating activities after 10 p.m., and to routinely go to bed at 12 a.m., as well as keep a journal of his sleep (hours, quality, evening activities) and a fatigue symptom diary. He returned 2 weeks later as requested, with slight improvements in his night sleep and daytime fatigue. Laboratory studies then showed: hemoglobin 12.8, WBC 10K lymphocytes 32%, monocytes 13%, eosinophils 4%, no atypical lymphocytes, and heterophile antibody was negative. He continued to slowly improve over the next month and discontinued his afternoon naps.

Chronic Fatigue

Prolonged fatigue is continual fatigue for at least 2 months, but not more than 6 months. Chronic fatigue is continual fatigue that lasts 6 months or more. Chronic fatigue syndrome (CFS) can be a cause of long-term fatigue, but since more adults than adolescents have this, and adolescents often do not meet all criteria for CFS, it is called chronic fatigue of adolescents (CFA), not CFS.

Causes of Fatigue

1. Lack of sleep and poor sleep habits are the most common causes.
2. Too many activities, the stress of planning, and time management issues: school, homework, extracurricular activities, social life and romance all contribute and need to be prioritized.
3. Emotional causes: depression, substance abuse, eating disorders.
4. Physical causes: medicine side effects, anemia, thyroid dysfunction, pregnancy, chronic infection (including infectious mononucleosis), cancers, as well as inflammatory bowel, autoimmune and neuromuscular diseases.
5. Chronic fatigue of adolescents.

True sleep disorders and diagnosable hypersomnia are not common, but adolescents need 7–9 hours sleep per night; this decreases with age. Many adolescents with poor sleep habits do not get this during weekdays. If they lived by their natural circadian rhythm, they would stay up late at night and would wake later than adults. Experts have observed teens in sleep labs, measured their melatonin levels, and found that nature makes it hard to get adolescents out of bed at an early hour. Their body clocks run on a schedule incompatible with the common early-to-rise routine. Natural rhythms cause most teens to prefer to sleep from 2 a.m. to noon rather than from 11 p.m. to 7 a.m. Unfortunately, most secondary schools have not adjusted to this, yet sleep researchers would prefer adolescents start school at 10 a.m. It has been shown that even a modest delay in school start time as small as a half hour is associated with significant improvements in alertness, mood and health [Owens, 2010].

The clinician can share some of this information with families, and counsel how to manage mornings: Do as much as possible the night before (pack up schoolwork, shower, lay out clothes, prepare lunch, lay out breakfast supplies) to ensure that he or she can spend as much time as possible in bed. Avoid doing anything stimulating before bedtime — exercising, playing violent video games, eating or drinking foods containing caffeine. Caffeine drinks can ruin sleep. Make sure he or she has a regular bedtime routine that is predictable and will invite sleepiness. Bedrooms and study rooms should not be the same, and neither should be filled with multi-tasking media technology.

Chronic fatigue syndrome in adolescents (CFA) is not the same as in adults (CFS). Often, it begins after a viral illness, with persistent symptoms and continual fatigue. Exhaustion occurs after mild physical activity or a stressor. Fatigue may become so bad that the patient cannot do many activities, cannot concentrate or attend school.

Adequate sleep does not improve it. Headaches, sore throats, adenopathy, arthralgias and myalgias can occur, as well as abdominal pains, fevers, nausea, vomiting, diarrhea, and anorexia. Many adolescents with CFA may need a few years to recover completely. About a third have poor recovery and continue with some disability.

Evaluation

The history must differentiate between weakness from fatigue and weakness from easy fatigability. A detailed sleep history is necessary. Ask questions about caffeine and substance abuse. Determine if there was a preceding viral illness. Inquire about fever, weight loss or gain, rashes, gastrointestinal symptoms, and for females, a menstrual history. Take a family history, social history, and evaluate stressors. A fatigue checklist may be helpful. Include a mental status examination.

The physical examination should note general appearance, skin color and pallor, thyroid gland, adenopathy, abdominal masses, hepatosplenomegaly, and signs of eating disorders. Screening laboratory tests can include a complete blood count, mono tests, thyroid stimulating hormone (TSH), erythrocyte sedimentation rate and urinalysis. Further evaluation to rule out organic causes of fatigue may also include Epstein-Barr virus (EBV) titers, antinuclear antibody (ANA), TB testing, and possibly, stool for ova and parasites if anemia, eosinophilia, or a history of certain travel exists. Most imaging studies are usually of limited value.

Management

With appropriate history, a complete physical examination, and some screening labs, begin by having the patient adjust sleep habits, if indicated, and keep both a sleep and symptom diary. This confirms that the symptoms are credible and worthy of evaluation. When a clear diagnosis causing the fatigue is made, then specific intervention is possible. When there is a diagnosis of CFA, then the symptom diary descriptions of daily fatigue or activity levels can help the clinician and family monitor change or improvement. Parents must be cautioned about assigning blame and expressing disapproval of their apparently "lazy" adolescent. A supportive, well-informed family will work with the clinician to assist the adolescent patient over the expected duration of the disease, which may vary. Appropriate progressive exercise or activity planning, as well as supportive psychotherapy, is often necessary. Stress management training and antidepressant medication can be helpful. Work with the adolescent's school to be sure that the patient receives appropriate support services and class limitations as necessary. Additional measures can be taken for infectious mononucleosis as discussed below.

Mononucleosis & EB-Virus

Infectious mononucleosis (IM) is common but can be a severe infection during adolescence. It is caused by the Epstein-Barr virus (EBV). Typically, fever, pharyngitis, lymphadenopathy, hepatosplenomegaly, and then prolonged fatigue are symptoms, but there are other mono-like syndromes caused by different infections such as CMV, toxoplasmosis, hepatitis-A, herpesvirus, adenovirus, rubella and HIV.

By adulthood, nearly everybody has antibodies to EBV. Many children have had asymptomatic EBV infection by mid-childhood, but when the infection occurs in adolescence or young adulthood, it is more often symptomatic. The incidence of IM among college students is higher than that among teenagers. Infection often occurs from contact with oral secretions, and it has been called "the kissing disease". The incubation period for EBV is about a month.

IM is a common, benign, self-limited disease in 99% of adolescents. Usually, a viral prodrome appears, with gradual onset of headache, chills, sweating, malaise, anorexia, and inability to concentrate. Fever is often present and may occur for a month, with high afternoon or evening peaks. The usual symptoms are the triad of prolonged fever, sore throat (unresponsive to antibiotics), and lymphadenopathy. Instead of usual anterior cervical lymph nodes, in IM they are usually the posterior cervical nodes. Other physical findings include periorbital edema, splenomegaly, and palatal petechiae. Splenomegaly can be palpated on deep inspiration in only half of patients, usually in the second or third week of illness. The rash of IM is usually faint and seen on the upper chest and neck. Streptococcal throat infection occurs as frequently in IM patients as in others with pharyngitis, which is about 20%.

Diagnosis of Infectious Mononucleosis

- Tonsillopharyngitis in 85% of patients.
- Fever, sore throat, malaise.
- Lymphadenopathy, mostly posterior cervical.
- Splenomegaly.
- Periorbital edema.
- Soft palate petechiae.
- Atypical lymphocytosis: > 10% total WBCs, > 1000/mm^3 total.
- Lymphocytosis: > 50% in differential count, > 4500/mm^3 total.
- Positive monospot or heterophile antibody or Epstein-Barr virus antibody test.
- Mildly elevated liver function tests (in 85% of patients).

There is proliferation of reactive 'T'-cells, the "atypical lymphocytes" seen in peripheral blood. A blood count usually shows 50% lymphocytes and monocytes, with

10% or more atypical lymphocytes. Liver function tests/enzymes are mildly elevated in 85% of patients and usually return to normal within 1 month. Extreme atypical lymphocytosis may even suggest leukemia. The heterophile test may be negative, and the disease is somewhat milder in younger patients and in those with negative heterophile titers. Some serology, monospot or heterophile antibody, or specific EBV antibody tests should eventually become positive. Mono-like syndromes caused by other agents often have a negative heterophile test, yet show atypical lymphocytes. IM is dynamic, with changing laboratory tests; the monospot is a rapid slide test that assesses the presence of heterophile antibody — which is not specific for EBV infection. This antibody is made against many different antigens; it is a qualitative test, as is the monospot, which is fast and 98% accurate. The rise of heterophile titers in IM varies. Neither one is specific for EBV, nor do they always turn positive. In teenagers, the heterophile response usually peaks in the second week of the illness. The monospot test should be done in the second week of illness, not immediately. The most common cause of heterophile-negative or monospot-negative IM is still EBV infection. The best way to make a retrospective IM diagnosis is by showing increasing specific EBV tests.

The most worrisome complication of IM is rupture of the spleen, yet it is very rare — usually occurring in males. Sometimes, a ruptured spleen is the clinical presentation and occurs usually during the second or third week of the illness. Neurologic complications can be severe in some cases. The leading cause of death in IM is neurologic complications, with most presenting as meningoencephalitis. Airway obstruction from extreme tonsil enlargement, glottic edema, or peritonsillar abscess can occur. Estimated case fatality rate for IM is only 1 in 3000.

Management

Treatment of IM may include antibiotics only if a throat test for group A Streptococcus is positive. Steroids may be used for 5–7 days (with no need to taper) only if there is impending airway obstruction. Decreased levels of T-helper and T-suppressor cells occur in those treated with steroids. Antiviral agents typically are without success. Bed rest and limited activity as tolerated are recommended during the febrile period. Later, patients can determine their own individual level of activity. Antipyretics or analgesics can be used for relief of fever, sore throat, and headache. In the presence of splenomegaly, for about a month, limit strenuous exercise, contact sports, and any activity creating increased intra-abdominal pressure or possible abdominal trauma. Almost all patients who take amoxicillin or ampicillin (and some on plain penicillin) will experience a florid, maculopapular rash. It is not an allergy; it is safe to finish the medicine. This usually starts almost a week after beginning the antibiotic (as opposed to acute allergic reactions occurring within 2–4 days and including hives).

Psychosomatic Illnesses

An adolescent patient with a psychosomatic condition is one of the most difficult challenges in adolescent medicine. Few disorders call for such advanced diagnostic and management skills; psychosomatic illnesses require skill in the "art" of medicine. An inaccurate diagnosis can result in false-positive, repeated and/or expensive tests, "doctor-shopping," and sometimes even unnecessary surgery. Psychosomatic illness is a diagnosis of inclusion as well as exclusion. The mind and body are not separate. All illnesses have a psychological and a physiologic component. Three foundations for the diagnosis of a psychosomatic disorder are:

1. Organic disease is ruled out.
2. Psychosocial dysfunction is present.
3. When the psychosocial dysfunction decreases and self-regulation occurs, the symptoms of the illness should improve.

Catherine is a Caucasian female who had an early history of Oppositional Defiant Disorder when referred to psychiatry at age 7 with problems at school and temper tantrums, which reportedly began with bullying by boys and no intervention by the school. She had school-based counseling in elementary school for tantrums, peer problems, and oppositional behavior. For ongoing headaches at age 10, a non-contrast CT of head was normal. Psychiatric referral at age 13 revealed trouble-making friends and feeling classmates hate her. She began to have intermittent migraines with emesis and abdominal pain. Symptom diaries were kept intermittently. Further workup at age 14 included a CBC with lymphocytes 37%; monocytes 7%; eosinophils 7%, ESR = 29; an EBV capsid-Quant POS; nuclear IgG qual POS, capsid IgM NEG; with an interpretation: past EBV infection. Serum for B. Burgdorferi AB was negative (done for Lyme Disease exposure by father's history). Stool culture revealed no *Salmonella*, *Shigella* or *Campylobacter*. Heterophile antibody was negative, and ANA nuclear antibody was negative. Urinalysis, TSH, and Free T4 were all normal, as well as a number of other tests. Then, she presented with headache and fever, had a complete series of tests of spinal fluid that were negative, but the influenza A PCR was positive, and influenza B PCR was negative.

Later, her mother reported she had trouble learning, concentrating and with relationships with peers. The patient was absent most of the school year in grade 9 for illness. Upper abdominal pains continued, and an abdominal ultrasound revealed a small gallbladder polyp with non-calcified stone, but was otherwise normal. A HIDA scan later showed the ejection fraction of the gallbladder to be decreased, with a value of 21%, but otherwise normal examination with prompt visualization of the gallbladder, common bile duct and small bowel. The diagnosis of chronic cholecystitis was made and she then had surgery for biliary dyskinesia; her gall bladder was removed. With a few months of improvement, she had few abdominal symptoms until age 15, when she reported left flank pain with bloody urine, and a workup including CT of the abdomen and pelvis was normal. She continued with abdominal pain, nausea, vomiting (without HA), and she was then seen by a gastroenterologist who did LFTs and full abdominal evaluation with negative lab tests. The diagnosis made was functional bowel/colonic spasm. She had trials of ranitidine, promethazine, and topamax with little improvement.

She later had another psychiatric evaluation for multiple somatic complaints that prevented her from attending school for months (stomach problems, vomiting daily, migraine headaches). When asked in session about any upsetting events prior to her illness this school year, she told about her dog dying from being accidentally dragged by the family car, then she cried, held her ears and refused to respond further. Further family history obtained: She lives with her mother and father, and her father is now being treated for bipolar disorder, gets migraines, and is on a medical retirement for physical and emotional problems. Her mother pressures her for high grades. Mental status: immature 15-year-old female who clutched her stomach and looked ill. She was lethargic and appeared dependent and passive. Her demeanor and school history were opposed to her desire to attend college and become a veterinarian. She had difficulty speaking for herself. Mood appeared anxious; affect was depressed. Thinking was coherent, and insight was poor. She denied suicidal and homicidal ideation, plan, or intent. Psychiatric assessment was: Long-term difficulty with social interactions including peer relationships and oppositional behavior, opposition related to school, and school avoidance from illness. Probable behavioral/emotional component is reinforced by parents. Patient has difficulty expressing feelings. Current diagnosis: adjustment disorder with mixed emotional features; parent-child problem; undifferentiated somatoform disorder; psychosocial and environmental problems (moderate problems with primary support group; problems related to the social environment; educational problems; other psychosocial and environmental problems). Challenges to treatment: apparent family dysfunction; patient's/parent's expectations for resolution of the problem; school attendance. Plan: family therapy and school consultation. Behavioral structure will be implemented by the school and followed through by parents.

An adolescent with a psychosomatic disorder is not usually aware of the psychosocial distress or psycho-emotional component. If the patient could identify and manage stressors, subconscious somatization would probably not occur. If he or she could adequately express feelings of guilt, depression, anxiety or frustration, then the chest pains or headaches may not have developed. However, in most cultures and societies, physical illness is more acceptable than poor coping or emotional distress.

About 25% of women and 15% of men report sexual abuse as children or teenagers. Adolescents (and children) with a history of physical or sexual abuse are far more likely to develop somatic complaints or a psychosomatic disorder. In a study of 3000 elementary schoolchildren who had physical complaints, those who were bullied were 2–3 times more likely to have headaches or abdominal pains. Because of teenage drug use, early sexual intercourse, and the influence of the media, today's adolescents need coping strategies earlier in their development.

Stress and Symptoms

All adolescents worry about dating, boyfriends or girlfriends, sex, parents (their illnesses, arguments, divorce), teachers, bad grades, and problems with siblings. Male adolescents often worry about eating, popularity and trouble with the law, while female adolescents worry more about menstrual periods and deaths of family members or friends. Research has demonstrated correlations between levels of stress and the incidence of colds and flu, asthma and allergic rhinitis, the durations of other illnesses and hospitalizations, as well as frequency of injuries. The field of psychoneuroimmunology has identified the links between the central nervous system, the peripheral nervous system, hormones, and the immune system. This provides a possible mechanism for how poor control of organic diseases such as asthma and diabetes can be worsened by psychological and psychosomatic issues.

Somatic symptoms are often a learned behavior. At a young age, children in some families learn that somatic complaints are more acceptable than expressed feelings. Children or teens with somatic symptoms often have been exposed to a family member who has a chronic physical illness.

The Triad of Anger, Fear, and Stress — then Reactive Depression

Adolescents may deal with problems by the innate *fight or flight response*, and this will create the unpleasant emotions of anger and fear. If they react this way most of the time, they get angry or afraid, and usually lose battles; they get frustrated, then eventually become sad and depressed or develop psychosomatic symptoms. This stress response is often the root of disease. The biological mechanisms of stress, distress, depression, and disease are a physiological continuum. The outward signs of psychosomatic symptoms and depression differ by age and gender: "Women get sad, and men get mad." Men more often show anger, frustration and discontent; women more frequently experience worry, fear, and tears.

The *triad of anger, fear, and stress (then depression)* is our basic set of *inherited survival emotions* and the common emotional denominator for personal problems. When adolescents get angry and aggressive toward others too often, or if they continually fear and retreat from others, then they can become upset with losing and may feel depressed or develop somatic symptoms. Over-reliance on fight or flight brings on the emotions of anger, fear, and stress/depression, which come from aggression, flight, and frustration. People get angry, fearful, or depressed because we are psychophysiologically constructed to feel these ways — it allowed our ancestors to survive harsh conditions.

Anger, fear, and depression had survival value, and are chemically controlled in the brain. Even though we have the human alternative choice to aggression and flight — that is, verbal problem solving — we will still *feel* the emotions programmed within us, no matter what we do. There are times we will feel afraid and angry from our inherited psychophysiology, but we can assertively interact with others. That is when one has the best chance of getting at least a part of what he or she wants, and the automatic anger and fear is less likely. If adolescents are frustrated with something they cannot change, if they fail to use the innate verbal ability to cope with something they could change, then they are more likely to feel emotionally depressed or develop psychosomatic symptoms.

Neurophysiologic coping mechanisms of anger-aggression, fear-flight, stress, depression-withdrawal and psychosomatic symptoms are not themselves signs of poor coping (or being at fault); they are just not much use to us. They rarely work or help situations. Most conflicts and problems come from dealing with others, and our primitive coping responses are rarely successful in comparison to our uniquely human coping abilities of verbal assertive problem-solving and learned self-regulation. These skills are reflected in the development of self-identity as a basic task of adolescence.

Anger-fight and fear-flight stress reactions actually interfere with cognitive coping ability. When angry, afraid or under high stress, an adolescent's primitive lower brain centers will automatically shut down much of the operation of the new higher brain centers; the blood supply is rerouted away from the brain and gut to muscles to prepare for action. The higher problem-solving brain is now inhibited from processing information. Adolescents do not think so clearly then and hence, they make mistakes.

Most adolescents are trained as children to be responsive to manipulative emotional control. These psychological puppet strings are attached through learned feelings of nervousness and anxiety, shame and guilt, and by controls over their assertiveness.

This protected them from danger as children, but as adolescents and adults, these are used by others to get them to do what *they* want. Learning assertiveness skills allow adolescents to eliminate some of these learned emotions in coping with other people. It takes practice to become aware of and in control of one's beliefs that allow others to manipulate them. In time and with practice, these verbal skills are easily learned for everyday situations that enable adolescents to enforce their rights as human beings and not be manipulated by others.

Making Psychosomatic Diagnoses

There is no one test for psychosomatic illness. Somatization is defined as the occurrence of one or more physical complaints for which appropriate medical evaluation reveals no explanatory physical pathology or pathophysiologic mechanism, or, when physical pathology is present, the physical complaints or resulting impairment are grossly in excess of what would be expected from the known physical findings. Adolescents who somatize often have associated psychological symptoms. There may be a history of early or chronic trauma resulting in "neurological vigilance". The physical concern or complaint may be a means to get help from an adult or clinician, and the physical complaint is often the stressor.

In making a diagnosis, the clinician should follow and reassess the patient frequently, rather than ordering an immediate "shotgun" battery of tests. Too often, a medical workup is done, and when it is negative, the adolescent is sent to a psychiatrist. Most patients and families dislike this, and it is not therapeutic; the message is, "The problem is in your head, and you need a psychiatrist to fix it". Personal validation is important to adolescents with psychosomatic concerns who will appreciate the clinician's genuine interest. In evaluating an adolescent who may have a psychosomatic disorder, the clinician must maintain a high index of suspicion, especially if there is chronic abdominal pain, chest pain, or headaches. However, even good practitioners cannot often determine a source of stress or anxiety at the first visit, even when a thorough history is taken.

Factors That Should Alert the Clinician to a Psychosomatic Diagnosis
- History of multiple visits to different physicians.
- Previous history of multiple somatic complaints.
- Dysfunction in adolescent development — especially family, peers, school.
- A manipulative and "enmeshed" family, where feelings are not expressed, or where parents avoid conflict.
- Presence of a "role model" in the family who has chronic or recurring symptoms.
- Reaction to the symptoms is disproportionate to actual disability.

Patients and families may be reluctant to accept the diagnosis of a psychosomatic disorder. To avoid this reaction, the clinician may refer to the problem as "stress-related" instead of using the term "psychosomatic". Family members will usually agree that it is better to have a stress-related disorder than an organic disease (stress-related abdominal pains vs ulcerative colitis; stress headaches vs brain tumor). To facilitate acceptance of stress-related problems, use known analogies like "exam diarrhea" or the tension headache at the end of a hard day. Do the organic and psychological workups simultaneously, and reassure that further organic testing can always be done in the future if needed.

Some Diffuse Symptoms of Stress-Related Problems
- Fatigue
- Chest pain
- Abdominal pain or Indigestion
- Headache
- Diarrhea
- Back pain
- Neck pain
- Nervousness, feeling shaky inside
- Trembling
- Heart pounding or racing
- Tightness in the chest
- Breathlessness
- Hot or cold spells
- Faintness or dizziness
- Feeling suddenly scared for no reason
- Feelings of impending doom
- Lump in the throat or choking sensation
- Frequent urination
- Amenorrhea
- Insomnia

Some specific somatoform conditions include: undifferentiated somatoform disorder (with a wide range of physical complaints, sometimes exaggerated and/or with an air of indifference), conversion disorder (a single motor or sensory symptom often associated with a stressor), hypochondriasis (preoccupation and fear of a serious but non-existent medical problem), body dysmorphic disorder (a preoccupation with an imagined flaw or slight defect in appearance or body structure), and pain disorder (disruptive pain in one or more anatomic sites where psychological factors have had a critical role in development or maintenance of the pain).

Chronic Chest Pain

Chronic chest pain in teenagers is common. The symptom is recurrent for over 6 months in about one-quarter of adolescents with such pains. Etiologic diagnoses are usually benign, but most teenagers seriously worry about their chest pains; over half fear heart disease, and 1 in 8 worry about cancer. On examination, palpate the costochondral junctions or compress the ribs to elicit costochondritis. Hyperventilation is a difficult diagnosis to make because patients are unaware of their breathing behavior. While few are aware of breathing too fast and too shallowly, half report anxiety, paresthesias, or light-headedness. A basic chest pain workup could include a chest X-ray and sometimes an electrocardiogram (ECG) if indicated by history of the symptoms; of particular concern is chest pain or syncope with exercise, or chest pain that awakes the adolescent from sleep.

Chest Pain Etiologies in Adolescents
- 35% Musculoskeletal (including trauma, costochondritis and precordial catch syndrome).
- 30% Idiopathic (benign — substernal vascular spasm, etc.).
- 25% Psychosomatic (includes hyperventilation).
- 10% Miscellaneous (breast abnormalities, esophagitis, cardiac (about 2%), and respiratory — including pneumothorax).

> Abdominal pain, headache and hypertension are included in this chapter on psychosomatic illnesses because the common treatment approaches to recurrent functional abdominal pain, most common headaches, and benign hypertension include lifestyle modifications similar to those recommended for most psychosomatic illnesses.

Chronic Abdominal Pain

Chronic abdominal pain is common in adolescents, and less than 10% will have organic lesions. Therefore, 90% is likely to be psychosomatic in origin. The incidence of inflammatory bowel disease is quite low.

Common Organic Causes of Chronic Abdominal Pain
1. Constipation: the most common cause of chronic, organic abdominal pain, and easily diagnosable with a careful history and physical examination.

2. Lactase deficiency: a history of symptoms associated with milk intolerance. Those with lactose malabsorption may have chronic abdominal pain and some diarrhea. Lactase deficiency is more common among Asian, Mexican-American, Mediterranean, Native American, and African-American populations, and lowest in Northern Europeans.

3. Irritable bowel syndrome (IBS): functional bowel disorder: diagnosis requires recurrent pain and a dysfunctional pattern of elimination such as diarrhea, constipation, or alternating both (organic but psychologically modulated).

4. Gastroesophageal reflux or gastritis: usually responds rapidly to anti-reflux or antacid medications.

A basic chronic abdominal pain workup should include a complete blood count (CBC), erythrocyte sedimentation rate, urinalysis, a pregnancy test for females, and sometimes, stools for occult blood as well as ova and parasite tests. If chronic abdominal pains are "crampy", then a trial of an antispasmodic may help make the diagnosis. Sexually active female adolescents should also be tested for sexually transmitted diseases (STDs) and have a bimanual pelvic exam because of the possibility of subacute or chronic pelvic inflammatory disease. Abdominal pain is also covered in Chapter 7, as it is often related to STDs, PID and UTIs.

Headache

Headaches are extremely common during childhood and adolescence, with incidences as high as 50%. Migraine headaches affect up to 10% of adolescents, but 20% of adolescents have experienced a migraine headache. Nearly 5% of teens suffer from frequent or severe headaches.

Lisa is a 15-year-old inexpressive, overweight Asian female with headaches (HA) three times a month for 6 months. History revealed bi-parietal and bi-temporal pain with level 5 of 10; no vomiting or nausea. Between HAs, she is completely fine. "No stresses" per mom, and bio-psycho-social screening is negative for stressors or specific signs of depression. No medicines taken before this visit; acetaminophen often helps. Sometimes, she has morning HAs with pain level 7 of 10, or after school when the weather is hot (pain = 7). HAs are not progressive. Her mother has a history of HAs twice a month, but not migraines. Plan: keep a complete headache diary.

Two weeks later: HAs are "the same". HA present 2 out of 3 days; pain level averages 6, but varies; lately has been occipital but moves around; it lasts 15–60 minutes, off and on; she sometimes gets an aura. No food or action known to cause it. Education and handout given on migraines and migraine triggers.

Two weeks later: HAs now shorter duration: 10–40 minutes, then gone. Nothing can stop it; occurs 5 out of 7 days; pain = 7; now occipital and throbbing, but had a bi-temporal episode. Now on loratadine in mornings and afternoons which seems to have helped some. Plan: continue diary; patient watched educational video on Relaxation Response, with a plan to teach focused imagery next visit.

One week later: Headaches only 10–15 minute duration, and pain level now 6–7 of 10. A 17-minute focused imagery relaxation exercise was trained, and she took home an audio program of another 10-minute relaxation exercise.

One week later: Had done focused imagery five times before dinners over past 1 week, as well as the 10-minute relaxation exercise before breakfast, six times over the past 1 week. HAs only occurred twice since last visit. They were only 10 minutes in duration, and pain level was 4 of 10. No further acetaminophen was used.

Two weeks later: Doing better. Focused imagery is done in the evenings only, five times in last 2 weeks, but 10-minute relaxation exercise was done 10 times in the mornings. She had only three mild headaches in the last 2 weeks which lasted 10 minutes (none at school). Plan: 5-minute evening relaxation exercise and 1-minute exercise in the mornings.

Two weeks later: Only one HA since last visit; pain level 3. She was 60% convinced treatment/relaxation practice resolved it. She felt it was 40% school pressure related, and that there is a 50% chance it is stress-related.

Although the fear of missing an early brain tumor is common among practitioners, brain tumors occur very rarely in adolescence — an incidence of three cases per 100,000. Even with available brain scans, the best screening test is still a good neurological exam — it will identify 94% of patients with brain tumors. About 80% of adolescents with headaches from brain tumors will manifest neurological or vision problems within 2 months of the beginning of headaches. Two-thirds of them are awakened from sleep with headaches, and three-fourths have vomiting.

Classifications of Headache
- Frequency: acute, chronic, mixed.
- Incidence: recurrent, progressive, non-progressive.
- Type: migraine, tension, organic.

Differential Diagnosis of Headaches

Acute, non-recurrent headaches are most often caused by upper respiratory infections, viral syndromes, and acute sinusitis, while most chronic headaches in adolescents are migraine or tension-type headaches. A *chronic progressive headache*, a headache that increases in frequency and/or severity over time, is the least common but most worrisome pattern. It is the most likely to represent serious underlying pathology, such as a brain tumor or other causes of increased intracranial pressure. Prompt and aggressive evaluation is required to rule out serious intracranial pathology. *Chronic non-progressive* headaches are most frequently encountered. Neuroimaging is rarely indicated in the presence of a completely normal neurologic examination. A *mixed* headache pattern may be chronic daily tension-type headaches with intermittent acute migraines.

Differential Diagnosis of Acute Headache
- Infection: flu/colds, sinusitis, meningitis, encephalitis, or intracranial abscess toxins, including environmental toxins, medications (e.g. stimulants), or illicit substances.
- Hypertension.
- Dental problem.
- First migraine headache.
- Trauma, concussion or postconcussive state.
- Intracranial or subarachnoid hemorrhage.
- Aneurysm, cerebrovascular accident, other vascular problem.

Chronic Progressive Headache

Chronic progressive headache is the most likely headache pattern to be associated with severe pathology, such as a brain tumor, abscess, or other intracranial mass lesion. Hydrocephalus, vascular malformations, aneurysms, vasculitis, and chronic or intermittent subarachnoid hemorrhage can also cause this headache pattern. Idiopathic intracranial hypertension (pseudotumor cerebri) is characterized by elevated cerebrospinal fluid (CSF) pressure in the absence of a mass lesion or obstruction of CSF flow; patients may present with generalized headache, sixth and third cranial nerve palsies and loss of vision; neuroimaging is normal. Posttraumatic and postconcussive headaches are common and may follow even mild head injuries. They may be progressive or non-progressive, persisting up to 3–6 months following the injury and resolving gradually; they may have migrainous and/or tension-type features.

Headaches from brain tumor usually have at least one of these:
1. Recent onset (within 4 months).
2. Presence of neurological abnormality, often ocular findings (papilledema, decreased acuity, or loss of vision).
3. Persistent vomiting.
4. Increasing severity.
5. Pain awakening patient from sleep.

Chronic Non-Progressive Headache

Chronic non-progressive headache is the most common adolescent headache, and is most often a migraine or tension-type headache. *Tension headaches* are the most common type of chronic non-progressive headache. The pain is typically mild-to-moderate, and patients can usually function during the headache. The pain may be dull or squeezing and located anywhere in the head. Adolescents may have headaches with features of both vascular and tension-type headache symptoms, confusing the diagnosis. *Migraines* are characterized by a specific constellation of symptoms: pain is usually unilateral frontotemporal, but may be bilateral especially in younger patients. There may be an aura, nausea, vomiting, photophobia or phonophobia. A recurrent pattern is necessary for the diagnosis of migraine; the first migraine headache is in the differential diagnosis of acute headache. A menstrual migraine occurs during at least two-thirds of menstrual cycles.

Analgesic withdrawal headache often follows analgesic overuse for chronic daily headache. It may occur following the withdrawal of any analgesic that has been used for several weeks. Other causes of chronic non-progressive headache:

1. Cluster headache — rare in adolescents.
2. Temporomandibular joint disorders with jaw pain and tenderness.
3. Posttraumatic headache.
4. Refractive error is a rare cause of chronic headache if no eye pain exists.

Evaluation

The clinician must balance doing too few and too many diagnostic tests. Chronic headaches may be associated with a 10% incidence of abnormal sinus films, and patients may respond to medical treatment for sinusitis. Brain scans should be reserved for those patients with specific neurological signs or symptoms or those who have life-threatening or acutely reversible conditions. Depressed adolescents may show poor school performance, sleep difficulties, or other depressive equivalents discussed in Chapter 6.

History to Obtain for Evaluation for Headache
- Headache pattern: timing, frequency, and progression of headaches.
- Quality (throbbing, dull aching, "squeezing", etc.) and severity.
- Location of pain in the head.
- Associated pain (eyes, neck, shoulders, tooth, jaw, face).
- Associated symptoms: nausea/vomiting, photophobia or other visual disturbance, phonophobia, neurologic symptoms.
- Headaches vary in quality and/or severity?
- Preceded by an aura or prodrome?
- Worse with physical activity (e.g. climbing stairs, walking)?
- Symptoms of systemic illness and/or infection: fever, neck stiffness, malaise, myalgia, weight loss, fatigue.
- Triggers: stress, fatigue, caffeine use and/or withdrawal, alcohol, chocolate, foods, menstruation.
- Affecting school attendance, peer activities, or work?
- Family history of migraine.
- Mental health history/symptoms.
- Psychosocial stressors.
- Medication use history: doses, frequency of use, efficacy, prescription, non-prescription.
- Use and abuse of illicit substances.
- Symptoms of elevated intracranial pressure (ICP): nausea/vomiting, early morning wakening with pain, ataxia, mental status change, other neurological signs.
- History of: head trauma, seizure, hydrocephalus, presence of ventriculo-peritoneal shunt, other neurological problems.

Physical examination includes:
- Vital signs: fever, hypertension.
- HEENT: Tenderness of head, sinuses, temporomandibular joint.
- Sharp disc margins on fundoscopic exam A papilledema.
- Restricted or painful jaw opening.
- Dental caries or tenderness of teeth.
- Nuchal rigidity, tenderness or spasm of neck muscles.
- Complete neurological examination.

Testing and neuroimaging: Often no ancillary testing is necessary, particularly in the evaluation of chronic non-progressive headache. Neuroimaging is rarely useful in the evaluation of headache without objective neurological findings. Over 95% of adolescents with brain tumors have such findings. Scanning should be considered in a patient with chronic *progressive* headache.

Indications for Neuroimaging in Adolescent Headache
1. Posttraumatic headache.
2. Focal neurological symptoms or abnormal neurological exam.
3. Visual disturbance (other than photophobia).
4. Progressive symptoms.
5. Mental status changes.
6. Evidence of increased intracranial pressure.
7. Growth/pubertal arrest.

Having the patient keep a *headache diary* is most useful; headaches that occur only on schooldays or in certain situations will lead to an investigation of situational stressors. For all chronic non-progressive headaches, the headache diary is a very valuable evaluation tool, revealing triggers, patterns, and associations of which the patient was not previously aware.

Headache Diary Items
• How long did headache last?
• What were you doing? Possible triggers.
• Any vomiting? Other symptoms.
• How severe was the headache? 1–10 scale.
• Day of the week. If school day, did you stay home?

Management

When headaches are symptoms of a physical condition or systemic illness, treatment of the underlying condition is the therapy. Otherwise, lifestyle changes, including optimizing diet, hydration, exercise, and sleep patterns may play a critical role in headache management. Focus should be placed on increasing physical function rather than on eliminating pain. Consistent school attendance may be an appropriate specific goal for many adolescents.

Once serious pathology has been ruled out, either clinically or with appropriate testing and/or imaging studies, patients (and their parents) should be reassured that the provider knows the diagnosis and that it is treatable. Specific mention that brain tumor is not the cause of the headache can be particularly important. The importance of lifestyle changes must be emphasized: patients should eat regular meals, not skip breakfast, and reduce or eliminate caffeine intake. Any foods or food additives that are known to trigger migraines should be eliminated, but broad "elimination" diets are usually not helpful. Good hydration during activities should be maintained. Adequate sleep (7 hours or more a night) and good exercise habits are critical. More extensive counseling with a mental health provider may be useful to address underlying mood or anxiety symptoms, assist with stress management, and help the patient develop appropriate coping strategies. Such a referral may be desired for evaluation and treatment of an underlying mood or affective disorder and to assist with non-pharmacologic treatment strategies.

Other non-pharmacologic techniques and skills may be useful for headache, particularly by teaching an internal locus of control rather than the choice to take a drug. Self-hypnosis, biofeedback, and relaxation techniques described later in this chapter are all useful. A multidisciplinary team approach may be appropriate for treatment of chronic headaches, as with many other psychosomatic illnesses.

Medications

Nonspecific analgesics such as NSAIDs are often effective and should be used in appropriately high doses. Triptans are the mainstay of migraine treatment when nonspecific treatments are ineffective. Dihydroergotamine may be used in adolescents over age 18. Narcotic opioids should be avoided in the treatment of all adolescent headaches. Analgesic rebound headache can be avoided by limiting the use of medications to a maximum of three times a week. Abortive medications for migraine headache should be available both at school and at home so that treatment may be initiated as soon as possible at the onset of headache. Patients who experience migraine headaches two or more times a week, have severe and debilitating headaches, or have a poor response to abortive treatments may be candidates for daily prophylactic medication. Daily low-dose amitriptyline is widely used for treatment of migraine, tension-type headache, and analgesic rebound headache. The use of valproate and other antiepileptic drugs is increasing.

Medications Used for Prophylactic Therapy for Adolescent Migraine
- Amitriptyline, cyproheptadine.
- Propranolol (beta-blockers).
- Carbamazepine, valproic acid.
- Riboflavin (vitamin B_{12}).

The treatment of menstrual migraine may include oral contraceptive pills to reduce frequency, but are contraindicated in the treatment of migraine with focal neurologic symptoms. Patients with focal neurologic findings or headaches that are refractory to treatment should be referred to a neurologist. Referral to a specialist nearly always results in comprehensive testing to look for organic disease.

Hypertension

Adolescent hypertension is defined as systolic or diastolic blood pressure greater than the 95th percentile for age, height, and gender. Hypertension is classified as *primary* or *secondary*. Primary hypertension is more common in adolescents than in children partly because of the increasing prevalence of obesity. Underlying kidney disease is the most common cause of secondary hypertension. Most adolescents with hypertension are asymptomatic. During evaluation, confirm the diagnosis of hypertension by repeated measurements on multiple occasions with proper technique. Once an adolescent is found to have an elevated blood pressure (usually >140/90), multiple readings (at least three) should be done on different occasions before hypertension is diagnosed (unless severe and the patient has symptoms).

> Optimal BP measurement technique: The adolescent should rest for at least 5 minutes. The inner cuff bladder width should be approximately 40% of the mid-arm circumference; the bladder within the cuff should encircle at least 80% of the arm.

Once the diagnosis of hypertension is confirmed, the workup includes past medical history of: recurrent urinary tract infections or renal injury, headache, chest pain, dyspnia, rashes, arthritis, diet, weight loss and constitutional symptoms (including sweating, flushing, palpitations, muscle cramps, weakness, or constipation). A family history may indicate a hypertensive family (which tends to have higher blood pressures than a normotensive family), since inherited hypertension may show hypertension in other family members. A social history should look for use of medications and recreational drugs, tobacco, alcohol and anabolic steroids.

The physical examination should include pulses checked in all four extremities. Blood pressure is measured in both an upper and a lower extremity to rule out coarctation of the aorta. Measure height, weight and calculate body mass index (BMI). The physical examination should evaluate thyroid, body habitus (e.g. buffalo hump) and skin changes or cafe au lait spots. The fundoscopic examination may rule out arteriolar narrowing or arteriovenous thickening. The cardiovascular examination looks for tachycardia, arrhythmias, cardiomegaly, murmurs, and signs of early heart failure. Examinations for carotid and abdominal bruits should be done. A thorough neurologic examination should be performed.

Differential Diagnosis of Hypertension

- Psychological stressors: most common.
- Renal: glomerulonephritis, DM nephropathy, trauma, recurrent UTIs, VCU reflux, polycystic kidney disease, chronic renal failure, neuroblastoma, Wilms tumor.
- Substances: high salt or caffeine intake, steroids, oral contraceptives, stimulant medications, decongestants, nicotine, illicit drugs such as amphetamine, PCP, cocaine.

- Vascular: coarctation of the aorta, renal artery stenosis (Williams syndrome, neurofibromatosis), arteritis (HSP).
- Endocrine: thyroid disease, CAH-Cushing syndrome, hyperaldosteronism, Hyper-PTH, pheochromocytoma.
- Other conditions: increased intracranial pressure, Guillain-barre, familial dysautonomia.

Laboratory testing and diagnostic evaluation of moderate and severe hypertension should start with certain screening tests for all patients diagnosed with hypertension: complete blood count (CBC), electrolytes, glucose, blood urea nitrogen (BUN), creatinine, calcium, uric acid, cholesterol, along with a urinalysis, urine culture, and often, a renal ultrasound. Other tests to be considered, depending on clinical suspicion and level of response to treatment, include: C3, C4, ANA, plasma rennin, urine catecholamines, plasma and urinary steroids including aldosterone, thyroid function tests, pregnancy test for females, echocardiogram (not an EEG) as a test to rule out left ventricular hypertrophy, a renal Doppler study, and sometimes, computed tomography (CT) scan of the abdomen and pelvis.

Management

The goal is to keep the systolic and diastolic blood pressure less than the 95th percentile for the patient's age, height, and gender. For secondary hypertension, the underlying cause is specifically treated. Higher goals are set for patients with chronic renal disease and diabetes since blood pressure below the 90th percentile provides a renal protective benefit. Patients should be followed every 2 months, but more frequently if they have severe or uncontrolled hypertension.

Lifestyle modifications including dietary interventions, weight reduction, and exercise constitute the first approach to treatment. These lifestyle modifications are effective in controlling blood pressure from all causes. Reduced salt diets help decrease blood pressure. Regular daily exercise has proven beneficial — a half hour of brisk walking daily can decrease blood pressure by 10 mm Hg. In obese adolescents, weight loss of only 5% can decrease blood pressure. Stopping tobacco, cutting down alcohol intake, and a low fat diet all help reduce blood pressure. Sports and physical activity in adolescents with hypertension should not be restricted. In those with severe hypertension, competitive sports and isometric exercises (i.e. weight training) may be restricted. Patients should be allowed to participate in aerobic physical activities, as it may help reduce blood pressure.

When lifestyle modification alone is insufficient, medications used in adolescents are similar to those used in the adult population. The choice of medications depends on the cause of the hypertension, the contraindications, side effects, and medication compliance.

Common Antihypertensive Medications for Adolescents
- Atenolol 1–2 mg/kg/day up to 100 mg/day, or Propranolol 1–4 mg/kg/day up to 640 mg/day.
- Hydrochlorothiazide 1–3 mg/kg/day up to 50 mg/day.
- Lasix 1–6 mg/kg/day.
- Lisinopril 0.07–0.6 mg/kg/day up to 40 mg/day.

General Management of Psychosomatic Symptoms

Improvement of psychosomatic conditions may require use of a number of standard as well as "adjunct" treatment approaches, which are often used simultaneously.

Behavioral and Environmental Interventions

The process of keeping a *symptom diary* itself is often therapeutic and frequently facilitates an adolescent's better understanding of the symptoms. When the stress can be rehearsed or anticipated, the adolescent is less likely to feel distress. Patients can learn two different coping strategies: "emotional-reaction-focused" (handling feelings and reactions without changing the stress), and "problem-focused" (changing the stress). The stress response can be managed and mitigated by a number of different approaches, and some are more practical than others for certain individuals.

Interventions to Help Control the Stress Response
- Positive self-indulgence.
- Physical exercise.
- A healthy diet.
- Time management.
- Keeping a sense of proportion.
- Nurturing relationships.
- Family and social support.
- Changing self-talk.
- Understanding and accepting the stress.
- Anticipating the stress.
- Rehearsing a response to the stress.
- Changing the stressful situation or environment.
- Assertiveness training and empowerment skills training.

- Controlled breathing.
- Relaxation response training and conditioning practice.
- Self-hypnosis, biofeedback, other self-regulation training.

Changing the problem and the environment may be difficult, but sometimes a minor change can help, such as speaking with a troubling teacher, changing a class or arranging for a tutor. If there is physical or sexual abuse, relocating the teenager may be required. Family therapy by a mental health professional and other family-oriented interventions may be needed for severe symptoms, non-response to treatment and non-compliance with medical advice.

Counseling and Psychotherapy

The primary care provider can usually provide the necessary information and counseling to adolescents about psychosomatic symptoms and causes, and rarely does treatment require referral for specialized psychotherapy from a mental health professional. Visits to a primary care provider tend to be shorter, easily tolerated by adolescents and more supportive, rather than insight-oriented. When psychotropic medications are needed, then a mental health professional may become involved, but the primary care provider continues to offer the most education about and ongoing monitoring of symptoms, progress, and expectations.

A primary care clinician is often the best person to do such counseling, which is not psychotherapy *per se*. When patients or families will not see a psychotherapist, a clinician with a long-term relationship with the patient has much to offer. Counseling can focus on the source of stress and discuss alternative ways of coping with it. To eliminate a symptom, the patient may require another strategy that is more efficient for dealing with the main stressor. Severe disturbances and anxiety should probably have an assessment by an adolescent psychiatrist. Anti-anxiety medications and SSRIs are often prescribed in consultation with a psychiatrist, unless the physician is experienced in psychopharmacology.

Relaxation Training, Self-Hypnosis, Biofeedback and Other Adjunct Interventions

Relaxation training and hypnosis are appropriate for highly motivated adolescents who learn to identify tension and relax the involved muscles. Relaxation training, guided imagery, and self-hypnosis all accomplish this to different degrees. They are particularly useful for teens who have chronic tension headaches or migraines.

Biofeedback can be used for adolescents who have many somatic symptoms or who are not insightful or verbal. It is very useful in families with denial of the psychosomatic aspect of symptoms but want control over them. Various approaches systematically rehearse self-regulation. Adolescents with chest pains, chronic headaches, or abdominal pains find this very helpful. There are highly advanced learning techniques for self-regulation training using brainwave biofeedback which is the state of the art.

Applied psychophysiology is the study of interrelationships between the mind and the body used in clinical, educational, sports, business, military, and many other areas. These clinical training techniques are called behavioral medicine. With the technology of computer-assisted self-regulation and biofeedback, changes in the personal physiology enter the awareness and are used to voluntarily monitor and modify the emotional climate (the neurochemistry) and the neurophysiological state. Training empowers patients by developing the ability to perceive with clearer focus, to better process information, and provides more choices including the freedom to choose resilient behavior. It is well known that intellectual information alone does not have the power to train the autonomic network.

Suboptimal physiological functioning occurs at various times of stress, and it is common to not realize when some physiological system is not functioning at the best level for a particular situation. Example: Many people get headaches because they keep muscles in their jaws too tense for too long (either because they do not realize their jaw muscles are tense, or because they do not habitually relax their muscles after a need for tension is over).

Behavioral Medicine Learning Techniques Used Clinically

Biofeedback (body self-regulation) helps patients
1. recognize how a physiological system is functioning.
2. learn a habit of controlling the system so it works optimally.

Self-Hypnosis (mind self-regulation) helps patients
1. develop intention and focus on a goal.
2. think and act in a more relaxed and deliberate manner.

There are a number of physiological signals typically recorded in biofeedback training, such as respiration, heart rate, muscle tension (surface electromyogram), sweating (galvanic skin response), skin temperature (near surface blood flow), and brainwaves (electroencephalogram). Brainwave biofeedback is frequently called "neurotherapy". These specific brain-based training techniques can help the adolescent brain learn to make normal transitions between brainwave states, rather than being habitually stuck in one state, often causing psychosomatic symptoms. They teach a permanent tool, allowing brain operations to become more flexible so that behaviors can change.

Using currently available technology, the results of change of psychophysiological processes and issues can occur with precision and speed unmatched by older approaches. Some of the newer technologies available for internal body self-regulation and development of appropriate arousal levels include: heart rate variability training, audio-visual entrainment, autonomic biofeedback, and brainwave biofeedback (including Beta/SMR and Alpha/Theta training). Such brain enhancement training technology assists in reaching individual goals, and can create efficiency, intuition, focus, endurance, and emotional resilience.

Self-hypnosis enhances the thoughts and functional focus. As a technique, it is an alternative state of awareness in which an individual develops focused concentration on an idea or image, with the expressed purpose of maximizing potential function and/or reducing or resolving a symptom or problem.

Self-Hypnosis Principles
1. Attention: concentrate on one idea, brings that idea toward realization.
2. Imagination: a very powerful subconscious tool.
3. Emotion: highly effective for creating change — particularly when combined with imagination.
4. Repetition of suggestion/affirmation: an important strategy for permanent improvement.

Self-hypnosis can be used as a "Change Agent". The steps of the process are: relaxation → changed perception/sensory experience → new imagery → emotion → changed cognition/meaning → changed conscious awareness → changed behavior → successful changes. When biofeedback technology and self-hypnosis are used in combination, they allow individuals to accelerate the process of self-regulation, higher awareness, and optimal performance. However, brain training technology and neuro-integration training is not magical or instantly transformative. They require the same kind of work as traditional long-term mental approaches, and ongoing personal practice of new skills and paradigms. Other complementary therapies such as acupuncture may also be particularly useful for some adolescents with psychosomatic illness.

Summary

Adolescents with psychosomatic illness usually present with organic symptoms, such as headaches, chest pain, or abdominal pains, rather than psychological symptoms. Psychosomatic pain hurts as much as organic pain. The psychological basis of the illness is rarely clear on the first office visit. The workup of psychosomatic illness should include the organic as well as the psychological components *simultaneously*. The extensiveness of an organic workup will vary, depending on symptoms. Remember: "When you hear hoof-beats, think of horses, not zebras". Consultation by an organ-system subspecialist may result in extensive and expensive testing; he/she will usually do the maximum testing available to rule out organic illness in the specialty.

In patients or families that are uncomfortable with a diagnosis of a psychosomatic illness, the finding of a "stress-related condition" should nonetheless be preferable over finding a significant organic disease. Advocate a "care versus cure" rehabilitative approach, which encourages return to usual activities and responsibilities even if symptoms persist. A rehabilitative team may include the clinician, family, school, psychotherapist, pain specialist, and other complementary health providers. As the symptoms take time to resolve, stay vigilant for potential diagnoses that were not initially obvious. The clinician will want to arrange frequent visits to monitor progress and guide the team to work together to address the evolving needs and concerns of the adolescent.

Suggested Readings and Bibliography

Anbar RD. (2003). Self-hypnosis for anxiety associated with severe asthma: A case report. *BMC Pediatr*, 3, p. 7.

Annequin D, Tourniaire B, Massiou H. (2000). Migraine and headache in childhood and adolescence, *Pediatr Clin North Am, 47*, pp. 617–631.

Benson H, Klipper MZ. (2000). *The Relaxation Response*. (Harper Collins, New York).

Blanchard EB, Radnitz CL, Evans DD, *et al.* (1986). Psychological comparisons of irritable bowel syndrome to chronic tension and migraine headache and nonpatient controls. *Biofeedback Self Regul*, 11, pp. 221–230.

Campo JV, Fritsch SL. (1994). Somatization in children and adolescents. *J Am Acad Child Adolesc Psychiatry*, 33, pp. 1223–1235.

Cavanaugh RM Jr. (2002). Evaluating adolescents with fatigue: ever get tired of it? *Pediatr Rev*, 23, pp. 337–348.

Chiarioni G, Palsson OS, Whitehead WE. (2008). Hypnosis and upper digestive function and disease. *World J Gastroenterol*, 14, pp. 6276–6284.

Chong Tong Mun. (1966). Psychosomatic medicine and hypnosis. *Am J Clin Hypn*, 8, pp. 173–177.

Gaylord SA, Whitehead WE, Coble RS, *et al.* (2009). Mindfulness for irritable bowel syndrome: protocol development for a controlled clinical trial. *BMC Complement Altern Med*, 9, p. 24.

Gill AC, Dosen A, Ziegler JB. (2004). Chronic fatigue syndrome in adolescents: a follow-up study. *Arch Pediatr Adolesc Med*, 158, pp. 225–229.

Hammond DC (ed). (1990). *Handbook of Hypnotic Suggestions and Metaphors*. (W. W. Norton & Company, USA).

Hammond DC. (2001). Treatment of chronic fatigue with neurofeedback and self-hypnosis. *NeuroRehabilitation*, 16, pp. 295–300.

Hyams JS. (2004). Irritable bowel syndrome, functional dyspepsia, and functional abdominal pain syndrome, *Adolesc Med Clin*, 15, pp. 1–15.

James LC, Folen RA. (1996). EEG biofeedback as a treatment for chronic fatigue syndrome: a controlled case report. *Behav Med*, 22, pp. 77–81.

Jones JF, Nisenbaum R, Solomon L, *et al.* (2004). Chronic fatigue syndrome and other fatiguing illnesses in adolescents: a population-based study. *J Adolesc Health*, 35, pp. 34–40.

Kinsman S. (2004). Caring for the adolescent with somatic concerns, *Adolescent Health Update*, 16, pp. 1–9.

Kohli R, Li BU. (2004). Differential diagnosis of recurrent abdominal pain: new considerations. *Pediatr Ann*, 33, pp. 113–122.

Lehmann D, Lang W, Debruyne P. (1976). Controlled EEG alpha feedback training in normals and headache patients, German [(author's transl)] *Arch Psychiatry Nervenrk*, 221, pp. 331–343.

Livingston R. (1992). Somatization, conversion and related disorders. In: McAnarney E, Kreipe R, Orr D, Comerci G (eds), *Textbook of Adolescent Medicine*, pp. 1080–1089 (WB Saunders Co., Philadelphia).

Mattulich L, Paperny D. (2008). *Journey to Awareness and Beyond, with Modern Technology and Ancient Wisdom.* (Xlibris Corporation, Bloomington). ISBN-13: 978-1436344647.

McKenzie R, Ehrisman W, Montgomery PS, Barnes RH. (1974). The treatment of headache by means of electroencephalographic biofeedback. *Headache*, 13, pp. 164–172.

Millman RP, Working Group on Sleepiness in Adolescents/Young Adults, AAP Committee on Adolescence. (2005). Excessive sleepiness in adolescents and young adults: causes, consequences, and treatment strategies. *Pediatrics*, 115, pp. 1774–1786.

Owens J, Belon K, Moss P. (2010). Impact of delaying school start time on adolescent sleep, mood, and behavior. *Arch Pediatr Adolesc Med*, 164, pp. 608–614.

Owens TR. (2001). Chest pain in the adolescent. *Adolesc Med*, 12, pp. 95–104.

Reeve A, Strasburger V. (1992). Basic principles of psychosomatic medicine in children and adolescents. In: Greydanus D, Wolraich M, (eds), *Behavioral Pediatrics*, pp. 352–366 (Springer-Verlag, New York).

Rice KM, Blanchard EB, Purcell M. (1993). Biofeedback treatments of generalized anxiety disorder: preliminary results. *Biofeedback Self Regul*, 18, pp. 93–105.

Samuels N. (2005). Integration of hypnosis with acupuncture: possible benefits and case examples. *Am J Clin Hypn*, 47, pp. 243–248.

Schneider CJ. (1987). Cost effectiveness of biofeedback and behavioral medicine treatments: a review of the literature. *Biofeedback Self Regul*, 12, pp. 71–92.

Shapiro BS. (1995). Treatment of chronic pain in children and adolescents. *Pediatr Ann*, 24, pp. 148–150, 153–156.

Silber TJ, Pao M. (2003). Somatization disorders in children and adolescents, *Pediatr Rev*, 24, pp. 255–264.

van Tilburg MA, Chitkara DK, Palsson OS, *et al.* (2009). Audio-recorded guided imagery treatment reduces functional abdominal pain in children: a pilot study. *Pediatrics*, 124, pp. e890–897.

Voit R, DeLaney M. (2003). *Hypnosis in Clinical Practice: Steps for Mastering Hypnotherapy.* (Routledge, USA).

Wright ME. (1966). Hypnotherapy and psychosomatic hypotheses. *Am J Clin Hypn*, 8, pp. 245–249.

Yucha C, Gilbert C, Association for Applied Psychophysiology and Biofeedback. (2008). *Evidence-Based Practice in Biofeedback and Neurofeedback*. (AAPB, Wheat Ridge).

Suggested Websites

Academy of Psychosomatic Medicine has as its central focus, patients with comorbid medical and psychiatric illness and the interaction between them: http://www.apm.org

American Society of Clinical Hypnosis, for licensed professionals who are trained and certified in clinical hypnosis: http://www.asch.net

Association for Applied Psychophysiology and Biofeedback, for professionals who are trained in biofeedback and neurotherapy: http://www.aapb.org

Biofeedback Certification International Alliance (formerly the Biofeedback Certification Institute of America, BCIA), board certification for specialists in various modalities of biofeedback, including neurofeedback: http://www.bcia.org

Chronic fatigue syndrome (CFS), also known as chronic fatigue and immune dysfunction syndrome (CFIDS): http://www.cfids.org

C h a p t e r 6

Psychology and Behavior

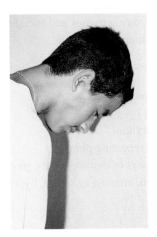

Life is largely a process of adaptation to the circumstances in which we exist. The secret of health and happiness lies in the successful adjustment to the ever-changing conditions on this globe. The penalties for failure in this great process are disease and unhappiness.　　　— Hans Selye

Overview

Two general principles of adolescent psychosocial development define the range of normal behavior in adolescence: 1. The transition from adolescence to adulthood is continuous and generally smooth. This period is generally not a time of "storm and stress". 2. Disruptive family conflict is not the norm. Mundane, everyday issues such as clothing, hairstyles, and chores are usual sources of conflict. See Chapter 2 for a complete discussion of normal adolescent psychosocial growth and development. With the exception of persistent childhood conditions, nearly all morbidity for teens and young adults results from behavioral choices caused by emotional, social and personal issues. Youths' behaviors that jeopardize their immediate and long-term health are often driven by psychological conditions.

The Psychiatric Mental Status Examination Includes Descriptions of

- Speech: rate, volume, articulation, coherence, and spontaneity with notation of abnormalities (e.g. perseveration, paucity of language).
- Thought processes: rate of thoughts, content of thoughts (e.g. logical vs illogical, tangential), abstract reasoning; and computation.
- Associations: loose, tangential, circumstantial, intact.
- Judgment: concerning everyday activities and social situations.
- Insight: concerning psychological condition.

and Evaluations of

- Orientation to time, place and person.
- Recent and remote memory.
- Attention span and concentration.
- Language: naming objects, repeating phrases.
- Fund of knowledge: awareness of current events, past history, vocabulary.
- Mood and affect: depression, anxiety, agitation, hypomania, lability.

Anxiety, Depression, Suicide

A stress reaction (as discussed in Chapter 5) followed by depression had survival value for our ancestors. Burn-out and depression cause us to slow down and do little except maintain necessary bodily functions (similar to hibernation). This was beneficial for putting up with harsh conditions in the environment — withdraw and retrench, conserve resources and energy — useful changes for survival until better times come along. Inversely, depression is now a sedentary disease, and physical exercise can actively improve the physiology of stress and depression. Controlled studies in Canada showed that physical exercise (defined as a half hour of movement that increased heart rate and caused some sweating) done four times a week was as effective as a selective serotonin reuptake inhibitor (SSRI) in relieving depression.

In today's society, reactive depression has little survival benefit. One way to lift depression is to cause (force) the adolescent to get back on his or her feet, moving again, and reconnect with positive life experiences, rather than to sit out the course of the depression without active management attempts. It is necessary to push oneself to get active to get out of depression. When he or she is doing poorly at work, school or socially, he or she must not repeat the past habit of fleeing from the situation by rehearsing the depressed feelings and withdrawing. Rather, finish the job at hand or continue the activity, even if the immediate feeling is that he or she does not want to. The adolescent will experience some discomfort, but with exercise, positive experiences and time, the psychological hibernation of depression often lifts.

Coping with Anger and Fear

Neurophysiologic coping mechanisms of anger-aggression, fear-flight, and depression-withdrawal themselves are not signs of poor coping (or being at fault); they are just not much use anymore. They rarely work or help the situations in which adolescents find themselves. Most conflicts and problems come from dealing with others, and our primitive responses are insignificant in comparison to our uniquely human coping ability of verbal assertive problem-solving and learned self-regulation. Anger-fight and fear-flight actually interfere with this cognitive coping ability. When angry or afraid, the adolescent's primitive lower brain centers will automatically shut down much of the operation of the new higher brain centers; the blood supply is actually rerouted away from the brain and gut to the muscles to prepare for action. The higher problem-solving brain is now inhibited from processing information, and the adolescent does not think so clearly — he or she makes mistakes. Adolescents need to remember, they usually have the right to declare a time-out to think things over!

A 19-year-old female had been having repeated occurrences of intense anxiety accompanied by frightening sensations of "pounding heart", chest pain, sweating, shortness of breath, and dizziness, along with a fear of dying or losing control. These would often occur for no particular reason. Recently, she was unable to drive alone over bridges or enter crowded department stores. Blood tests, physical exams, and an EKG of her heart had all been normal. She was diagnosed with panic disorder, and refused medication. Her treatment was cognitive behavioral therapy (CBT) with a psychologist, consisting of patient education, monitoring of her panic symptoms, breathing retraining, and cognitive restructuring of the catastrophic thinking associated with her panic symptoms; she was taught to identify and change anxious thoughts and predictions, and she also had exposure and desensitization to anxiety-provoking situations and physical sensations.

Exposure to feared sensations and situations was practiced several times a week until the fear decreased. CBT took her ten sessions. Approximately 2 months later, she returned with similar symptoms and was taught the specific Thought Field Therapy algorithm for panic and anxiety attacks which she practiced daily and used as needed. She has since managed her episodes by herself.

Anxiety

Anxiety is the most common psychological condition of adolescents, and few seek care for it. Anxiety (an emotion that occurs with perception or anticipation of loss or danger) creates the physiologic changes for "fight or flight", and when excessive or prolonged, this will cause functional impairment and an anxiety disorder. It begins with a trigger or stressor that causes the adolescent to exhibit avoidance/escape behaviors, or even begin a compulsive behavior. This maladaptive (but effective) behavior decreases anxiety temporarily, yet the reinforced behavior becomes a habit. Symptoms of anxiety may occur, or adolescents may have only somatic complaints (see Chapter 5). Anxiety disorder should be suspected in those with chronic or somatic complaints, especially when the severity of symptoms is greater than expected with the known stressor. Making the diagnosis of anxiety disorder requires significant distress and/or impairment of function.

Psychological Symptoms of Anxiety

- Feeling anxious, worried, scared, fearful, nervous, restless, or unsettled.
- Hypervigilance, hyperarousal, easily startled.
- A feeling of impending doom or disaster, a fear of dying.

Physical Symptoms of Anxiety

- Palpitations, increased heart rate.
- Short of breath, tachypnia, chest pains.
- Dizziness or fainting.
- Perspiration, skin flushing, or clamminess.
- Gastrointestinal problems.
- Feeling shaky.
- Paresthesias and "hysterical" symptoms.
  (also see list Some Diffuse Symptoms of Stress-Related Problems on page 104)

One in 15 adolescents has a generalized anxiety disorder, and 1 in 15 experiences social phobia in a year. About half that many have obsessive-compulsive disorder

(OCD). Over half of adolescents with anxiety can be diagnosed with two anxiety disorders, and a third actually have three. Anxiety disorders tend to run in families. Nearly half of adolescents with an anxiety disorder will have some form of depression. Anxiety symptoms may be the precursor of depression. Substance abuse commonly occurs as an attempt to self-medicate the anxiety.

A *generalized anxiety disorder* diagnosis requires more than 6 months of functional impairment, with no specific trigger or obvious stressor [Woo, 2008]. Specific, recurrent anxiety episodes or panic attacks (sometimes in specific situations, especially around unfamiliar people or possible scrutiny) come on quickly with slow resolution [Woo, 2008]. Some adolescents avoid social situations for fear of a panic attack around others (social phobia) [Woo, 2008]. Agoraphobia (being in a place with difficult escape) and other specific phobias (i.e. heights, flying, blood) are triggered by a specific object or situation. Those with OCD have obsessive thoughts and do compulsive actions, and 80% have both obsessions and compulsions [Woo, 2008]. Obsessions are recurrent thoughts of harm, cleanliness, concerns of contamination, and other impulses which are unreasonable but cause anxiety and need to be neutralized, such as making things symmetric. Compulsions are repetitive behaviors which reduce distress in response to obsessions, such as hand washing, re-checking, ordering and counting things. OCD is sometimes more effectively treated with clomipramine, rather than an SSRI like sertraline or fluvoxamine.

Posttraumatic stress disorder (PTSD) happens after an experience of actual or perceived possibility of death or harm. Common causes are physical or sexual abuse in childhood, personal assault, war, natural disasters, and deaths in the family. Almost half of sexually abused children and adolescents have PTSD. Reliving the trauma in dreams or flashbacks from certain stimuli bring on memories. The increased arousal causes hypervigilance, disturbed sleep, and problems focusing. The adolescent works hard to avoid the stimulus, then may become detached and emotionally numb. *Acute stress disorder* is similar to PTSD but occurs within a month of trauma and lasts up to a month.

Medical evaluation of anxiety signs and symptoms includes the mental status examination as well as a history of prescription medication use (steroids, asthma medications), over-the-counter medications (diet pills, caffeine), substances of abuse (amphetamine, cocaine), and possible withdrawal from substance use (alcohol, benzodiazepines, narcotics). The physical examination includes the thyroid gland and a neurologic examination. Continual tachycardia suggests possible hyperthyroidism. Uncommon differential (physical) diagnoses are hyperthyroid, pheochromocytoma, hypoglycemia, and cardiac arrhythmias. Random bouts of palpitations with anxiety disorder can be evaluated with cardiac monitoring. Except for the rare thyroid study, laboratory tests are usually not helpful.

It is important to give the patient reassurance that the symptoms are not dangerous, and inform family that they are real and not made up. A discussion of neurophysiologic coping mechanisms and the treatment approaches discussed in this chapter will be helpful. Energy psychology therapies (e.g. Thought Field Therapy) often produce remarkable improvements of phobias and other anxiety disorders [Sakai, Paperny, Mathews *et al.*, 2001]. Family therapy can help when the adolescent's symptoms have a major impact on family function. Family members may need to learn to respond correctly to the patient's symptoms and escape behaviors. Cognitive behavioral therapy or desensitization may be useful, and medications may also be necessary. Selective serotonin reuptake inhibitors (SSRIs) are used first for anxiety disorders; specific ones have been shown to be effective for treatment of specific anxiety and phobia diagnoses. SSRIs may take several weeks to show results; the dose must be titrated up for full efficacy. Routine use of anxiolytics should be avoided, but irregular use of benzodiazepines with a short half-life (i.e. lorazepam, alprazolam) may be used to help acute, severe symptoms and insomnia.

Depression and Bipolar Disorder

Depression and bipolar disorder in adolescents are now more common compared to a few decades ago. One in 5 adolescents will have an episode of major depression, which occurs twice as often for females than males. About three-quarters of depressed adolescents receive no treatment. Depressed adolescents may feel sad, like depressed adults, but often they only feel *irritable*, bored, negative, or apathetic. Depressive equivalents include school problems, substance abuse and acting out behavior. The outward signs of depression are different by age and gender. *"Women often get sad, but men get mad."* — Men show anger, frustration and may be easily upset; women may experience worry, fear, and little joy in life. There may be frequent somatic symptoms (see Chapter 5) and little or no understanding of how mood affects symptoms.

> A 17-year-old female with a vague history of sexual abuse as a child presented to the office with her mother, who complained that her daughter was irresponsible and lazy. She was sleeping about 11 hours every night, and always took a 2-hour "rest" during the day after returning from school. Her mother also said that the patient rarely talked to her (except for arguing) and had to be awakened every school morning. An uncle committed suicide, and the mother took fluoxetine a year ago; she divorced the patient's father 18 months prior. *Separately*, the patient reported not being able to concentrate on schoolwork for the last few months and has been feeling sad most of the time, saying, "Nothing is fun any more." She

denied serious previous suicide attempts and current thoughts of wanting to die, but said the last such thoughts were about 1 month ago. She was able to state that if she were to kill herself, it would be by "an overdose or something." The patient made a promise to call the clinician or the suicide helpline if she ever felt suicidal again. At school, she has two good friends, but she previously had more. She now has two failing and three passing grades in school, but denied alcohol or drug use. Her only exercise was walking home from school. On examination, her affect was flat and her mood included some tears at times. Judgment and thought were normal. The thyroid gland was normal, and she had several old linear scars 2 cm above her left wrist, but had no bruising or other skin lesions. The patient was made to understand that certain things will be necessary to do to feel better, including increased exercise, medication and counseling. She agreed to those, and a plan was made as to how all this will be presented to her mother. *Separately*, the mother was then counseled that depression is a specific medical condition creating her daughter's symptoms, and improvement requires support and not blame, as hard at that may be. She was made aware of the potential seriousness, and was asked to support her daughter when the three meet in a short while, where recommendations will be exercise, medication, and counseling. She required further explanation of medication issues. She was also warned to remove all potentially lethal medicines including acetaminophen from the house (which had only one floor and had no balcony). *Meeting together* with the patient and her mother, it was repeated that depression is a specific medical condition that is not anyone's fault, and that there is a three-part treatment, all of which is required for improvement. Negotiations for increased exercise included joining the mother at a fitness club three times a week and swimming twice a week. The patient and her mother were counseled in depth about starting fluoxetine at half dose for 2 weeks, then if no problems occur, to double the medication to 20 mg daily. Possible side effects were discussed, and the patient agreed to contact the clinician if there are any increased suicidal thoughts. Psychotherapy with a psychologist was arranged, and the mother agreed to work with the school counselor for academic assistance. A follow-up appointment was made for 3 weeks later.

An episode of *major depression* is 2 weeks or more of being depressed, bored, or irritable mood most of the time, with little interest in activities. A few of these must also be present:

1. Change in appetite or weight.
2. Insomnia or hypersomnia.

3. Fatigue or energy loss.
4. Psychomotor agitation or retardation.
5. Poor concentration and focus.
6. Feelings of worthlessness, hopelessness or guilt.
7. Frequent thoughts of death or suicide.

The symptoms must cause clinically significant distress, and must not be caused by substance abuse or another medical problem.

Nearly 1 in 10 adolescents have *dysthymia*, where depression symptoms are less intense and more chronic than those of major depression. For a year or more, the adolescent is depressed or irritable most of the time, along with some other depression symptoms. About 70% of these adolescents will have an episode of major depression. An *adjustment disorder with depression* can occur within 3 months of the presence of an identified stressor, but symptoms are more than what would be expected for the stressor and resolve within 6 months of the end of the stressor.

For adolescents with *mania* and *bipolar disorder*, there are depressive and manic symptoms which may occur in mixtures or cycle. A manic episode may include excessive pleasurable activities (and sometimes risky ones) like fast driving, hypersexualization, and money over-spending. There is a period of elevated or irritable mood for at least 1 week, and some of these symptoms will also be present:

1. Inflated self-esteem or grandiosity.
2. Talkative and distractible.
3. Racing thoughts.
4. Psychomotor agitation.
5. Decreased sleep.

About a third of adolescents with major depression will develop bipolar disorder within 5 years of the major depressive episode [Strober *et al.*, 1993]. A depressive episode is usually the first sign of bipolar disorder. Bipolar adolescents often have rapid cycling, with manic and depressive episodes a few days or even hours apart, and have frequent suicide attempts and completions.

Adolescents with mood disorders often have other conditions such as mild mental retardation, learning disorder, attention deficit disorder (ADD), oppositional-defiant disorder (ODD), or substance abuse (often the result of self-medicating depressive symptoms). The risk of experiencing a mood disorder increases with stress, family conflict, divorce, abuse or neglect, chronic illness, and a variety of social factors. When symptoms of a thought disorder (psychosis) occur in depression (found in 30% of patients with major depression), there is an increased risk of bipolar disorder later.

Medical evaluation for depression may include screening for anemia, vitamin B12 deficiency, mononucleosis, hyper- or hypothyroidism, a collagen-vascular disease such as lupus, and human immunodeficiency (HIV) infection. Chronic diseases such as diabetes, seizures, or asthma may facilitate depression, as can the use of corticosteroids, stimulants, neuroleptics, and hormonal contraceptives. The physical examination includes evaluation of weight, a mental status examination, the thyroid gland, scars from cutting arms or wrists, and signs of physical abuse or substance abuse. Except in the case of chronic disease or urine drug screening, laboratory studies are usually not useful except for evaluation of a physical finding or perhaps a screening test.

Depression and Suicide

"Suicide is not chosen; it happens when pain exceeds resources for coping with pain."

Suicide is the third leading cause of death for adolescents from 15–24 years old, and it is becoming more common, as is depression. Suicides among adolescents tripled from the 1950s to the 1990s. More die from suicide than from heart disease, cancer, AIDS, and birth defects combined. Possibly 1 in 5 secondary school students have considered suicide during the past year. Screening for depression can be done by interview, by questionnaire (see Chapter 1), and with the 21-item Beck Depression Inventory, where a score over 12 is worrisome. Whenever a depressed adolescent is identified, adequate evaluation must be done to assess suicide risk. Depressed adolescents should be queried about the cause of any recent injuries — to detect abuse as well as self-harming behaviors such as cutting, or a recent suicide attempt. Asking about suicidal feelings does not increase a patient's risk of suicidal behavior. When asked, suicidal adolescents are usually willing to express recent feelings to clinicians.

Depression History Items to Assess

- History of physical, sexual or emotional abuse.
- Family history of a suicide attempt or completion.
- Changes in peer group or peer relationships.
- Changes in appetite: usually decreasing but sometimes increasing.
- Changes in sleep patterns: too much or too little sleep.
- Changes in school behavior: failing grades, falling asleep in school.
- Parent-child conflict.
- Impulsiveness.
- Number of previous suicide attempts.
- Dysfunctional family unit: divorce, recent death, substance abuse.

Depression Screening Questions

- Are you mostly happy with the way things are going for you these days?
- Lately, have you often been sad, depressed or unhappy?
- During the past month, have you often felt hopeless?
- During the past month, have you felt really down, or like you have nothing to look forward to?
- Have you ever been to a counselor for help with your problems?
- Have you had any thoughts about not wanting to be alive?
- When some people get very sad or upset, they think about hurting or killing themselves; did you ever seriously think about doing that?

If a depressed adolescent is identified, a more extensive evaluation should include suicide screening. About 80% of successful suicides are by persons who have attempted suicide before. If the answer to any of the questions above is "yes", ask suicide screening questions.

Suicide Screening Questions

- Did you ever make a plan to kill yourself?
- Did you ever try to kill yourself, or hurt yourself in a way that you could die?
- In the last month, how often did you think about killing yourself?

Evaluation of Suicide Risk

Many "normal" adolescents, when routinely asked the suicide screening questions above, will surprise many interviewers. Adolescents most at risk for suicide are impulsive, or have sexual orientation issues, or are male. Males are more at risk since they use more lethal methods such as hanging or guns, and they are less likely to talk about their problems with adults or even friends, whereas females have more social support and more often express their feelings. Query the adolescent and the family members about the availability of lethal medications (e.g. acetaminophen), a convenient balcony from which to jump, or firearms at home.

Assess Factors That Increase Suicide Risk

- Gender (highest rates occur in males).
- Substance abuse (drugs or alcohol).
- Same-sex attraction or sexual activity, gender identity issues.
- Talking about death, death notes; giving away possessions.
- Rejection or neglect by others; feeling that nobody cares.

- Access to effective means of suicide, such as a balcony, gun or lethal medications including acetaminophen.
- Depressive equivalents: aberrant behaviors, psychosomatic symptoms, emotional outbursts, recurrent emotional lows.
- Depression items: low self- esteem, sadness; feelings of helplessness, hopelessness, or worthlessness.

If a suicidal adolescent is identified with the suicide screening questions, a more extensive evaluation should include assessment of the suicidal *intent* of the adolescent and the *lethality* of the method. Many adolescents do not know the lethality of a method they may have considered. The two most important questions to ask teens who are at risk for suicide are: 1. Are you planning to kill yourself? and 2. How would you kill yourself? After asking those two questions, you can then find out if they have support systems and resources in their lives when they feel suicidal.

Suicidal Intent and Lethality Assessment Questions (patient is interviewed alone)
- When was the last time you seriously thought of it? - (planned it).
- How would you do it? - (the method); if he/she says "I don't know" (you must get at least a hypothetical answer to this question), then ask: What way did you think you might do it?
- Before you did it, who could you call for help? (available support and resources); if he/she says "a friend" (referring to a peer), then ask: Is there an adult you could call?
- Do you have a friend or family member who tried to kill themselves, or did so?

Some worrisome methods are: "with my dad's gun" (indicates prior thought and specific plan), or "jumping off my balcony" or "hang myself" (common way males successfully commit suicide). Assess if there is a clear idea or a specific plan, and the lethality of the plan. When a teen asks about confidentiality, it is reasonable to tell the teen that information divulged about health is private unless there is an emergency, abuse or imminent danger to self. The parents of teens should also be interviewed to provide the history items regarding symptoms such as behavioral or school problems, and abnormal sleeping or eating patterns, as well as any expressed thoughts or threats of suicide.

Informing Parents and Family

If the patient is not an immediate danger to self, and family is present, then the parents are usually informed in terms of the clinician's "concerns for teen's feelings". The parent should usually first be privately informed of concern and need for follow-up.

Answer parent questions. Then, re-inform the parent with the teen present. If a parent is not present, contact a parent or family member based on lethality and imminent danger, or if the patient is of adult age, negotiate appropriate follow-up services. Other protective actions include:

1. Obtain promise to get help before hurting self; assess commitment to use resources including Crisis Helpline.
2. Assess availability of supervision before the patient is seen for mental health follow-up appointment.
3. Refer adolescent with limited suicidal intent to mental health specialist, and make the appointment before leaving the office.
4. Plan when and how parent/patient should follow-up or call if symptoms worsen or if crisis occurs (provide contact information).
5. Consider prescribing an SSRI (usually fluoxetine) immediately, rather than delaying until the mental health appointment.

Usually, the clinician can decide whether the adolescent is at ongoing risk for suicide. Immediate psychiatric evaluation for possible hospitalization is often necessary for suicidal adolescents who:

1. are still intent on suicide.
2. are those with significant previous suicide attempts.
3. are males
4. are severely depressed.
5. have significant substance abuse.
6. have considered a lethal method (e.g. firearm, hanging, jumping off a high place).
7. have no supportive environment or resources.

Intervention in a suicidal emergency, although rare, may require a psychiatrist to decide if outpatient or inpatient care is appropriate. If immediate treatment is needed for protection from imminent harm, immediate psychiatric consultation is sought regarding hospital admission. Most jurisdictions have a process whereby any licensed physician can request that an ambulance or the police transport such a patient to a psychiatric hospital for evaluation. Parents and/or guardians should be informed about actual suicidal behavior or significant levels of risk; confidentiality may be breached in the face of potential suicide and imminent harm.

Education of the Patient and Family

The patient (and family) must learn that depression is a common medical problem, that the hopeless feeling is treatable, and that the adolescent can feel better if they comply with all treatments. Make a crisis intervention plan, so that the family knows what to do if the adolescent becomes suicidal. Give resources ahead of time to access, should an emergency arise. In the absence of hospitalization, the family becomes responsible for ensuring the adolescent's safety at home. This includes supervision time together, and removing medications, poisons and firearms from the home. Since depressed or suicidal adolescents may find it difficult to follow treatment programs, they require a failsafe arrangement to monitor compliance with follow-up counseling. Explain that the primary health care provider will remain connected over time, and that in spite of referral to a mental health provider, the primary health care provider wants complete follow-up by the patient.

Parent and Family Education

- Limit access to a balcony, gun or lethal medications.
- Take statements seriously.
- Do not dismiss the adolescent's problems as unimportant (minimization).
- Do not give "easy advice" such as "Just be strong" or "You will get over this." (avoidance).
- Talk with the adolescent; really listen. Let them know they are not alone. Do not blame.
- Do not hesitate to get help for your adolescent and yourself.
- Depression is a treatable medical problem, with no stigma in getting help.

Treatment

The four necessary treatment components for depressed or suicidal adolescents are: 1. Counseling & psychotherapy, 2. Exercise & activities, 3. Medication, and 4. Monitoring. Patients and family should be informed that all four are required for the best outcome.

Psychotherapy such as cognitive-behavioral therapy (CBT) provided with an antidepressant produces improvement more than those treated with either therapy alone; those who only take an antidepressant may improve more than those who receive only CBT. CBT helps restructure the adolescent's self-critical thoughts and challenges negative perceptions. Plans are made for encouraging scheduled participation in enjoyable activities, increasing pleasurable activities, decreasing behaviors that reinforce the depression, and improving interpersonal skills. Other types of therapy may be necessary, such as general supportive therapy, interpersonal therapy, behavioral therapy and family therapy. Physical exercise (30 minutes of activity which increases heart rate and causes some sweating) done four times a week can be as effective as an antidepressant. It is important to encourage (or perhaps force) exercise and positive activities as part of self-care. Monitoring and close follow-up with the clinician is essential, even in patients who are referred to mental health specialists, since adolescents with depression have high rates of non-adherence to both mental health counseling and antidepressant medication.

Selective serotonin reuptake inhibitors (SSRIs) are the most commonly prescribed antidepressants for adolescents, since they are about 60% effective and have the fewest side effects. Side effects of SSRIs include gastrointestinal upset, agitation, sexual dysfunction, sedation, and sleep disturbances. They may cause hypomania or mania in some adolescents. Although the therapeutic effect of SSRIs usually takes 4–6 weeks to be noticeable, any side effects are usually obvious within the first few weeks. When an SSRI is prescribed, begin with half the usual dose (e.g. fluoxetine or citalopram 10 mg daily) for 1 week. If it is tolerated without side effects, it should be increased to the full dose (e.g. 20 mg). Adolescents may metabolize SSRIs faster than adults, so increased doses may be required for results; the dose can be increased every 4 weeks, to a maximum daily dose of fluoxetine 60 mg. Normally the medicine should be continued for at least 6–9 months when there is improvement.

If there is little response to treatment with one SSRI (occurs about half the time), or it is stopped due to side effects, it is recommended to try another SSRI. It is likely that one can be found which will benefit an adolescent clinically, and it is often necessary to try a few different ones before finding the one with no side effects and its best dose. Obviously, it may take time to find the best medication and the right dose, so patients and families need to be so informed. Paroxetine is often not recommended, and the lethality of overdose of tricyclic antidepressants limit that choice to specialists, particularly if the patient is suicidal, and dispensed medication quantity must be limited. Another class of antidepressants includes bupropion which is activating and useful for adolescents with depression, addiction and attention deficit hyperactivity disorder (ADHD), but is to be avoided in seizure and eating disorders. Antidepressants should not be prescribed to adolescents with bipolar disorder, and they should be used carefully in depressed adolescents with a family history of bipolar disorder. These patients are best treated by a mental health professional; mood stabilizers such as lithium, valproate, lamotrigine, and carbamazepine have all been used.

Recent publicized warnings about the risk of suicide for adolescents using antidepressant medications include SSRIs. Data are controversial, and studies so far have not definitively confirmed significant risk, but the "black box" warning about possible association of SSRIs with suicidal ideation in children and adolescents should be explained to patients and their parents or family. They should be told to notify the clinician if there is:

1. suicide attempt
2. increasing suicidal thoughts

3. more depression or anxiety symptoms
4. more panic attacks, agitation or impulsivity
5. new or more mania or hypomania symptoms.

The patient should be seen about 3 weeks after the prescription, more often as indicated based on risk, then regularly until the maintenance phase in reached. SSRI doses should be tapered before discontinuing the medicine; Discontinuation Syndrome occurs from too rapid discontinuation of SSRIs, manifesting crying spells, irritability, agitation, anxiety and flu-like symptoms including dizziness, headache and insomnia.

Primary care clinicians have a crucial role in the recognition and management of mental illnesses in adolescents. Most clinicians should be able to initiate treatment for mild-to-moderate depression without the aid of a mental health specialist, depending on the severity of symptoms, clarity of the diagnosis, and experience and comfort level of the provider.

Psychosis

Psychosis is an impaired ability to think, communicate, understand reality and respond emotionally. Specific symptoms include delusions, hallucinations, and disordered thought, speech and behavior. It can be caused by depression, bipolar disorder, substance abuse, certain medical conditions and schizophrenia. Schizophrenia occurs in 1% of the world's population. Early-onset schizophrenia has a peak age of onset in males at 18–25 years old, and for females it is 25–35 years old. Degrees of schizophrenia can be seen in schizoid and paranoid personality disorders. There are no diagnostic laboratory tests for schizophrenia but certain neuro-imaging scans show non-specific changes. When bipolar illness presents with psychosis, it is often misdiagnosed as schizophrenia. Combined variants of compulsion, thought, anxiety and other disorders (even Munchausen's Syndrome) can occur in adolescence [Paperny, 1980].

Violence, Conduct Disorder, and Abuse

Violence in adolescence has become a significant public health problem and a current health issue around the world. Homicide and suicide are leading causes of death among teenagers. In American secondary schools, a third of adolescents were in a physical fight in the previous year, and 1 in 6 carried a weapon to school in the last month; 1 in 10 boys have carried a gun to school. Adolescents are exposed to violent media worldwide, and violent attitudes and behavior are clearly influenced by watching violence on television. The proven association of media violence to aggressive behavior indicates that *violence is learned behavior*. Exposure to violence in the home and parental reliance on corporal punishment contribute to violence in youths. The majority of violent injuries involve adolescents who know each other and disagree, then fight. Assertiveness training and learning alternate nonviolent methods of coping with conflict and anger are crucial in violence prevention.

A clinical risk assessment of violence for an adolescent should include: how he or she copes with anger; if he or she ever carried a weapon; how safe he or she feels at home and at school; how likely he or she is to fight, and a history of ever being injured in a fight. Also inquire if a partner or date ever hit her or forced her to have sex, and also evaluate the adolescent as perpetrator: a history of injuring others in a fight, or if he ever hit her or forced a partner or date to have sex. The clinician's message should always be "No argument or disagreement ever justifies physical force." Provide appropriate counseling about how to recognize controlling or abusive relationships, and how to get out of a relationship that has intimate partner abuse. Some aggressive adolescents may have "masked depression". Gun safety is an important part of preventive counseling, and it is necessary to routinely ask if there is a gun in the home.

Bullying is a form of aggressive and violent behavior where adolescents intentionally harm, harass, or intimidate a victim. Four out of 10 children experience bullying, whether they watch it, they are a victim, or they are a bully. Bullying has devastating effects on everyone. The bully uses control and power over others. There are three types of bullying: 1. Physical, 2. Verbal, and 3. Relational, where the bullies try to convince their peers to exclude a person or group of people from their social connections. This happens online (cyberbullying) and via texting when bullies spread rumors about their victims or even embarrassing photos — the use of social manipulation and isolation of victims in schools. One child in 10 is regularly attacked by bullies, either verbally or physically. Most teenagers experience some harassment in their school at some time. Many do not report being bullied, and often experience anxiety, depression, or have school refusal. Statistics show that 1 in 4 bullies will have a criminal record before the age of 30. The intention of bullying is to put the victim in distress, and bullies seek power. They feel hurt inside and find it difficult to have empathy. Many bullies have been abused at home, or have otherwise been victims of abuse. Both victims and bullies have low self-esteem. Some victims have taken weapons to school and planned revenge. A useful tool for dealing with bullying is a program to mobilize the masses of students who are neither victims nor bullies to take action against bullying. These students have the potential to significantly reduce bullying simply by the way they react when they witness bullying incidents. Students can take action in many different ways by refusing to watch bullying and by reporting bullying incidents.

Oppositional defiant disorder (ODD) includes negative, hostile, or defiant behavior, with anger, arguments with authority figures, refusal to follow directions, and often shifting blame. There may be progression from ODD to conduct disorder (CD). ODD often occurs before CD and may be an early sign of CD. ODD is diagnosed when behavior is hostile and defiant for 6 months or longer. ODD can start in the preschool years, whereas CD generally appears when children are somewhat older. ODD is not diagnosed if CD is present.

Conduct disorder (CD) includes recurrent antisocial behavior, cruelty, running away, and truancy [Yiming, 2008]. Adolescents with CD may have aggressive behavior that harms or threatens to harm other people or animals, destructive behavior that damages or destroys property, lying or theft, and other serious violations of rules. Adolescents with CD repeatedly violate the personal or property rights of others and the basic expectations of society. Most adolescents with CD are probably reacting to negative events and situations in their lives. A diagnosis of CD is likely if the behavior continues for a period of 6 months or longer. CD can persist into antisocial personality disorder. Antisocial behavior and sociopathy are very hard to change after middle adolescence; therefore, CD must be identified and treated early.

Prostitution

Prostitution is a very self-destructive behavior. The isolation and danger of a fast street life have great potential for significant psychological and physical harm. Adolescents involved early in prostitution usually fail to acquire the educational and occupational skills necessary to succeed in the adult world. Many adolescents who are involved in prostitution are runaways who had poor relationships with parents, and sometimes parental abuse or neglect. Running away is clearly associated with entrance into juvenile prostitution. Physical and sexual abuse is very common in the early history and active street life of adolescents involved in prostitution. The youth street culture is often well-defined and provides a social support network as well as monetary resources for survival away from home [Deisher, 1975].

Unclear sexual identity and poor self-esteem may contribute to entrance into prostitution, which becomes a means of obtaining attention, feeling wanted and needed, and providing some sense of accomplishment. This positive reinforcement, perhaps the first positive input after a life of negative self-image and low self-esteem, can be a significant factor in a youth's entrance into prostitution. For many, the psychological harm can be measured by duration of exposure and gradually decreasing self-esteem and increasing negative self-image, as well as impact upon the future psychosexual relationships and later, sexual dysfunction. During this critical stage of adolescent growth and development, it contributes to a continued inability to cope with the adult world and its requirements. Over time, rehabilitation becomes progressively more difficult.

Approximately 65% of female adolescents involved in prostitution report having been raped, and 50% report having been pregnant. Mean age of first intercourse is about 12 years, and many such females have had experiences and conditioning that caused them to define their self-worth in sexual terms. From early childhood, these girls are rewarded for being cute, and they learn to use their attractiveness and sexuality to meet their emotional and later, physical needs.

For males involved in prostitution, the time for acquiring education, work habits, and job skills is passing (as for females too). Many become involved in criminal activities; most of their prostitution contacts are same-sex, the opposite of female prostitutes [Deisher, 1969]. Teenage male prostitutes can be divided into two groups that are nearly equal in number: those who self-identify as heterosexual, and those who self-identify as homosexual or bisexual. The former are usually more criminal and sociopathic in nature, and the latter are more likely to have left home because of persecution from his family or peers in school when they learned that he is homosexual; he has a tendency toward less violence.

The major mistake of health practitioners in managing adolescents involved in prostitution is to assume that because these youth are very sexually experienced, they have an understanding of sexuality, birth control, and sexually transmitted infections; this is rarely the case! Prevention and early intervention is the key, since it is extremely difficult to overcome reinforcement for this behavior and lifestyle once the excitement, money, drugs and alcohol, friends, and other "rewards" are experienced.

Maltreatment, Emotional and Physical Abuse

There is an association between the maltreatment, abuse and exploitation of adolescents and the predisposition to violent and other offending behavior [Paperny, Deisher, 1983]. Reported cases of abuse and maltreatment constitute only a small fraction of actual cases that are occurring (URSA, 1980). There are differences between the psychosocial dynamics involved in adolescent abuse and those of child abuse. Three types of physical abuse of adolescents exist: 1. Abuse beginning in childhood and continuing into adolescence, 2. Physical punishment and discipline from parents that increases significantly during adolescence, and 3. Physical punishment and abuse which has its onset in adolescence. In reviewing 70 cases of adolescent abuse, Lourie [1977] reported that most physical abuse begins when the youth reaches adolescence. Two behavioral and developmental tasks of adolescence — separation and control — lead to family conflict and ensuing abuse. Adolescent victims of abuse often run away from caretakers to avoid physical, sexual or emotional abuse. A study by Hopkins in 1970

[Berdie, 1977] of 100 detained youths showed that 77% reported they had been abused by a family member within the last 6 months; 84 had been abused as a child.

Runaways and adolescent offenders have frequent contact with violence and exploitation while on the streets and at home. They are often used for criminal purposes such as prostitution and other forms of trafficking in sex, drugs, and illicit activities. The most common factor in a predisposition to crime and delinquency is the child's tendency to identify himself with aggressive parents and pattern after their behavior. The association between abuse and violence has long been clear — the experience predisposes youth to use aggression as a means of problem-solving, accompanied by a lack of guilt or empathy for others, and a diminished ability to cope with stress in a practical way. About half of juvenile child molesters were either physically or sexually abused as children. [Deisher, Wenet, Paperny *et al.*, 1982]

Sexual Abuse

In many studies, about 1 in 6 females (and half as many males) report being forced to have sexual intercourse when they did not desire it. A variety of other unwanted sexual contacts are reported far more often than sexual intercourse. Some studies suggest 60% of teen mothers in the samples had unwanted/involuntary sexual experiences. Approximately 80% of runaways have been physically or sexually abused. The incidence of sexual abuse of males is probably higher than reported. About 90% of sexual abuse is committed by men, and usually it is a person known to the victim, such as a family member, friend of the family, or acquaintance. Sexual abuse usually occurs privately, often produces no physical signs, and is difficult to detect. Secrecy must end to stop most perpetrators. Psychosocial sequelae are the most significant complications of sexual abuse for both male and female victims. Two out of 3 victims manifest psychosocial symptoms, and many are sequelae of intrafamilial sexual contacts.

Molestation is noncoital sexual activity and may include viewing genitals, fondling breasts, or oral-genital contact. *Sexual assault* is any sexual contact with a non-consenting victim. *Rape* is when the penis enters (even the slightest amount) the victim's genitalia, by coercion or without consent; *statutory rape* is such sexual intercourse with a youth below the legal age of consent in the jurisdiction. *Incest* is sexual contact between individuals who are related and not able to legally marry, including parental figures who live in the home. *Sexual abuse* is any inappropriate sexual contact or exposure for her or his age, family role, or developmental level which violates law or social rules. This includes everything mentioned above as well as anal penetration (sodomy), sexual activity of an underage adolescent with an adult (or significantly older adolescent in some cases), as well as exploitation of underage adolescents in pornography.

Presentation of Sexual Abuse (behaviors not diagnostic, nor limited to sexual abuse)

- General statements implying unwanted sexual contact.
- Direct statements reporting sexual abuse.
- Sleep disturbances (e.g. nightmares, night terrors).
- Appetite disturbances/eating disorders.
- Neurotic or conduct disorders.
- Phobias, avoidance behaviors, new fears.
- Withdrawal, depression.
- Guilt, diminished self-esteem.
- Poor school performance.
- Inappropriately sexualized activities; sexual acting-out, promiscuity/prostitution.
- Excessive masturbation.
- Perpetration of sexual abuse upon others.
- Drug and alcohol use/abuse.
- Temper tantrums, aggressive behavior, acting-out.
- Self-mutilating behaviors (cutting, burning etc.)
- Runaway behavior/delinquency.
- Suicidal ideation/attempts.
- Hysterical or conversion reactions.
- Strained family relationships.
- Genital, urethral, or anal complaints.

Medical Signs of Sexual Abuse

- No physical findings are most common (only present < 10% of the time).
- Unusual aversive reaction to abdominal, pelvic, or genital exam.
- Psychosomatic complaints (particularly abdominal pain).
- Genital, urethral, anal lesions or trauma.
- Recurrent UTI.
- STD or pregnancy (especially in any adolescent under the age of consent).

Sexual abuse evaluation requires asking questions in this order for maximal validity:

1. When was the last time the sexual contact happened?
2. Do you sometimes still see this person?
3. Is it someone you live with now?
4. Who did it?
5. Describe the sexual contacts.

Computer-assisted screening and interviewing facilitates detection and evaluation of sexual abuse [Paperny *et al.*, 1988]. The immediate goals of a medical assessment are to identify injuries that require treatment, to screen for and preventively treat STIs, to evaluate and reduce the risk of pregnancy for females, and to document findings of forensic value. Detailed medical assessment is usually deferred until a comprehensive medico-legal forensic examination can be accomplished (preferably within 72 hours); it will complete the medical assessment as described, and also collect forensic evidence according to local standards to be used in a court of the local jurisdiction. The comprehensive medico-legal forensic examination of adolescents and young adults requires specialized approaches which are beyond the scope of this book [Gushurst C, Palusci V, 2010] and should be performed by an experienced forensic examiner.

Legal Reporting Issues

Most jurisdictions have formal child abuse reporting laws which apply to youths that have not reached legal adulthood. Agencies that are responsible for investigating allegations of child abuse vary, but usually include the police and some form of child protective services. The legal definition of abuse is derived from several sources, including: 1. reporting laws; 2. criminal laws (child endangerment statutes); and 3. juvenile law (which defines abuse, neglect, dependency, and may decide custody issues). Most reporting laws only require that you have "suspicions". It is usually not the clinician's job to prove abuse, only to report it. Other agencies are responsible for investigation and prosecution. If you are unsure whether or not to report, review the case with a representative of the mandated agency. The clinician should work with the reporting agency and the adolescent to develop a plan to provide for the adolescent's safety. Find out if there is a family member the teen feels comfortable calling for support, and who can provide or arrange for her/his physical safety.

Substance Use: Alcohol, Tobacco, Other Drug Use

Alcohol, tobacco and other drug use is ubiquitous for adolescents worldwide. Prevention and total abstinence from these is optimal, but more responsible use of alcohol needs to be promoted in many countries.

Tobacco Use

Tobacco use is probably the most preventable cause of disease and death in the world [Yiming, Kee, 2008]. It kills someone nearly *once per minute* — more than substance abuse, AIDS, accidents, suicide, homicide and cancers of the breast, prostate, and uterus *combined*. It increases risk of diabetes by up to three-fold, and is a major trigger for asthma. Adolescent smoking remains high (about 1 in 4 or 5), in spite of efforts to prevent and reduce it. About a third of adolescent smokers will later die from smoking-related pathology. Smoking is an addiction, not a habit; it is psychological, physical and behavioral, so effective treatment requires counseling, medication and active user participation.

Tobacco Prevention

Most smokers start smoking or become regular smokers during adolescence, and few people start smoking after adolescence. When a parent smokes, there is much more chance that a youth will become a smoker. Complete habituation to smoking takes about 2 years, when stopping then becomes significantly more difficult. Since it only takes 2 years for an adolescent to become a regular smoker, then the early years are crucial for prevention in younger teens and children.

No one is born with a craving to smoke. The first cigarette always tastes terrible, but people start smoking because it seems to be the accepted thing to do (a social norm — to be cool); because friends smoke (social pressure); because they are trying to act independent; because they want to feel grown up; because of curiosity; and because of pleasure (to calm nerves). Females often smoke to control weight, and it may also be related to low self-esteem. Preventive counseling about tobacco is important for clinicians to repeatedly address with all adolescents. Prevention should include discussion of the perception of cigarettes, family and peer smokers, and media suggesting social acceptability. Give each adolescent specific examples of resistance statements ("My doctor told me I can't smoke due to..."), and tell them to use them. Like a vital sign, ask tobacco use status at every patient visit. For those who do smoke, urge every adolescent tobacco user to quit, and evaluate readiness to quit.

Evaluation of Readiness to Quit
- *Pre-contemplation*: Not thinking about quitting.
- *Contemplation*: Thinking about quitting but not planning to quit in the near future.
- *Decision*: Planning to quit in immediate future.
- *Action*: Currently taking action to quit.
- *Maintenance*: Has maintained abstinence from use for an extended period of time.

Tobacco Cessation

Telephone support cessation programs have become a successful standard of care, and paying smokers to quit can boost success rates. Social support among smokers is strong, and the quitter must usually give up most social associations with friends who smoke, at least for a while. The adolescent will need to develop alternative social supports. Medications reduce withdrawal symptoms. If a smoker of more than 10 cigarettes a day is willing to make an attempt to quit, clinicians should prescribe bupropion and nicotine replacement therapy (gum, patch, others) when there is sincere desire to quit tobacco and a willingness to give up or limit exposure to smoking friends. Assist the patient in quitting, and help the patient quit with a plan. In preparation for quitting, instruct the patient to set a quit date within 2 weeks. He or she should tell family, friends, and coworkers about quitting, and request understanding and support.

Expect challenges to the planned quit attempt, particularly during the first few critical weeks, including nicotine withdrawal symptoms. Tobacco products are removed from the environment. Prior to quitting, the patient should avoid smoking in places where he or she spends a lot of time (e.g. work, home, car). Discuss challenges and triggers and how the patient will successfully overcome them. Identify what helped and what hurt in any previous quit attempts. Total abstinence is necessary: "Not even a single puff after the quit date." Alcohol can cause a relapse, so the patient should consider limiting or abstaining from alcohol while quitting. If there are other smokers in the adolescent's household, quitting is much more difficult, so the other smokers should plan to quit at the same time, or never smoke around them. Follow-up counseling during the first quit week is critical, and ongoing telephone follow-up programs are very effective. Adolescents should anticipate that most relapses are within 3 months after quitting.

It has been projected that if a one-pack per day smoker were to take the same daily cigarette money spent from age 20 to 60 and invest it in a stock market, he or she would be a millionaire at age 60! Adult smokers who quit smoking before age 50 cut their risk of dying in the next 15 years by 50%.

After Quitting:

1. Lung function improves after 2–12 weeks.
2. Heart disease risk drops to 1/2 that of a smoker after 1 year.
3. Stroke risk drops to that of a non-smoker after 5 years.
4. Lung cancer risk drops to 1/2 that of a smoker after 10 years.
5. Life span is increased 8–14 years.

Script of Tips for Successfully Stopping Smoking

You won't have to wait 15 years for tobacco to affect your health. It actually only takes 3 seconds. Three seconds after you take your first smoke, your heart beats faster, your blood pressure rises, carbon monoxide enters your blood, and cancer-causing chemicals spread throughout your body. Millions of people stop smoking every year. Not everyone can do it the first time, but most people *do* eventually succeed. Most smokers stop for good, after only a few tries. For young people, the *earlier* you stop, the *easier* it is. If you've been smoking heavily for a while, ask your health provider about Stop Smoking programs. You'd probably like to quit smoking, but you just don't think you can. Millions of people have done it, and so can you! First, you'll need to decide to put up with some discomfort, and then do these things:

- Choose a specific stop date, and stick with it.
- Tell your friends and family about your plan to quit.
- Throw away your tobacco in a special way.
- Brush your teeth often, and drink lots of water.
- Chew sugarless gum, celery sticks, carrots, or hard candy as a smoking substitute.
- Avoid things that are reminders of wanting a smoke, such as people who smoke.
- Find activities that make smoking difficult.
- Avoid places where smoking is allowed.
- Sit in non-smoking sections of restaurants.
- Reward yourself. Buy yourself things with the tobacco money you save.

Cravings and desire for tobacco are a normal part of withdrawal, but not much trouble after a few weeks. Most failures occur in the first week or two after stopping, when withdrawal symptoms are strongest and your body still wants nicotine. This will be your hardest time. Remember that *one* cigarette could start you smoking again. Alcohol or drugs will weaken your willpower. Once you've stopped, remember — *no* occasional smoking! Nicotine addiction comes back quickly. By stopping, you've done a great thing for yourself and your future. You *don't* have to be a smoker!

Alcohol Use

It is true that alcohol is the drug with the most serious consequences for adolescents worldwide, when considering morbidity and mortality from binge drinking and alcohol-related accidents. Millions of adolescents under age 18 years have alcohol problems. Heavy or even moderate alcohol drinking or binge drinking during adolescence can impair learning and memory and even interfere with physical development. The adolescent's hippocampus — important in learning and memory — is smaller among moderate and heavy drinkers. Drinking can lower estrogen, testosterone, growth hormone and bone density. Teenagers in Europe report drinking more frequently than teenagers in many other countries.

Alcohol Evaluation by *CRAFFT* Mnemonic (two or more "yes" answers suggest a serious problem with alcohol)

- Ever driven in a *Car* when someone (including yourself) was under the influence?
- Ever use alcohol to *Relax*?
- Ever use alcohol when *Alone*?
- Ever *Forget* things while using alcohol?
- Do *Family or Friends* tell you to cut down drinking?
- Ever gotten into *Trouble* while using alcohol?

In many countries, motor vehicle accidents related to driving under the influence of alcohol are a leading cause of death for this age group. Alcohol-related motor vehicle accidents cause adolescents six times more injuries and permanent disability than deaths. Clinicians are obligated to inform parents and young adolescent patients about the dangers of alcohol when driving as well as underage alcohol abuse. It is known that teens underestimate their drinking habits; they themselves do not think they drink excessively, but when quantified, many of them are in fact drinking heavily and often.

Psychoactive Substance Abuse

Many adolescents experiment with drugs during their teenage years; some are curious and try drugs (often marijuana), while others are addicted to dangerous drugs like cocaine and amphetamine. Alcohol, marijuana, and tobacco are all available to most adolescents worldwide [Song, 2008]. In evaluating adolescents, it is important to determine what kind of drugs they are using, and how often they use each specific drug or drugs, and if they feel a need to take drugs (cravings, family problems, etc.). This is especially important for potential teenage mothers who are taking addictive drugs or who are self-injecting users (at risk for HIV). Adolescents using drugs are at higher risk for other harmful behaviors that are associated with drug use (e.g. unsafe sex, alcohol abuse). These risky behaviors are often more dangerous in combination, with a greater synergistic effect (e.g. alcohol and sedatives).

Four Stages of Substance Abuse

1. *Experimental use*: Boys especially are most often experimenters with various mood-altering substances. Some may never go beyond the experimental stage,

but many of them will continue to experiment and become regular users. They most often use alcohol and marijuana in this stage and seek the mood swings that these drugs provide. The chemical use may stay at the social and recreational level. It is inappropriate to diagnose chemical dependency at this stage. Many adolescents have been inappropriately labeled as dependent when they are not.

2. *Regular use*: Using more does not, by itself, indicate dependency, but a pattern of regular use, coupled with some adverse behavioral changes, can show a definite tendency. What is important is why it is being used and any behavioral changes that occur as a result of the use. If teenagers have to lie to their parents about their companions and have to maintain other lies, they may be moving toward increased use.

3. *Problem use*: Preoccupation with drugs is a major indicator of a drug abuse problem. More time, energy and money are spent on being high and ensuring that the drug is available. Many of his or her daily activities include drug use, and the user accepts this as normal. Negative consequences such as problems with parents or police may suggest to the adolescent that it is time to cut down or quit, but there is continued use despite the harm which is obvious. Periods of abstinence do not last.

4. *Dependency*: By the time the user has reached a state of dependency, negative self-esteem and emotional turmoil require daily use of drugs. Abusers do not distinguish between normal and intoxicated behavior. Being high seems normal, and no argument can break through their chemically maintained delusion and emotional/physical addiction. This delusion persists even in the face of overwhelming evidence that his or her abuse is out of control and is physically and mentally suffocating. The abuser will continue to insist that there is no problem, that it is not out of control, and that he or she can quit at any time. However, there is physical tolerance to the drug, and there would probably be some withdrawal symptoms if stopped.

Substance abuse among adolescents causes mortality, morbidity and devastates families more than any other health problem in the world. Regular use of alcohol and drugs puts lives at risk. Often, parents are remarkably unaware of their adolescent's drug and alcohol use. A teenager's ability to deceive his or her parents often increases parents' denial about their child's drug use. There are many cultural, societal, social, personal, psychological, and biological risk factors that predispose an adolescent to drug abuse.

Psychiatric Conditions As Risk Factors For Substance Use Disorder

- Mood disorders such as major depression, dysthymia, and bipolar disorder.
- Anxiety disorders such as generalized anxiety disorder, social anxiety disorder, and posttraumatic stress disorder.
- Attention-Deficit/Hyperactivity Disorder (ADHD), and untreated ADHD (treated ADHD reduces the risk by 85%).
- Conduct disorder.
- Eating disorder: Bulimic patients have been found to have a greater risk for substance abuse than restrictive anorexics.
- Suicidal ideation: 70% of adolescents who complete suicide were drug and alcohol users.
- Schizophrenia: Patients with schizophrenia are at increased risk of abusing marijuana.

Protective Factors for Substance Use Disorder

- Stable family and home environment and strong parent-child bond.
- Personal motivation for achievement.
- Consistent parental supervision and discipline.
- Bonding to social institutions (e.g. religions, youth groups).
- Association with peers who have conservative attitudes.
- Exposure to early anti-drug messages.

Other Factors Associated with Substance Use

Cultural/societal

- Social norms favorable to drug use.
- Availability of drugs.
- Extreme economic deprivations.

Interpersonal

- Family alcohol and drug use and conflict.
- Maladaptive family management and parent personalities.
- Physical or sexual abuse.
- Stressful life events (i.e. relocation).
- Association with drug-using peers.

Psychobehavioral

- Psychopathology (depression, anxiety).
- Early and persistent behavior problem.
- Academic failure and little commitment to education.

- Alienation, rebelliousness, or antisocial personality.
- Sensation seeking and inability to delay gratification.

Biologic and Genetic
- Inherited tendency toward substance use.
- Psychological and physiological vulnerability to drug effects.

Clinicians need to become familiar with:

1. The most common drugs of abuse used by adolescents in their community.
2. The current use patterns of these substances by local adolescents.
3. The pharmacology, intoxicant effects, treatment withdrawal effects, and clinical treatment approaches.
4. Community treatment resources.

Methamphetamine Abuse

Methamphetamine ("Meth", "Ice") has been around for quite some time. Amphetamine use skyrocketed in the 1960s, and crystal methamphetamine became common in the 1990s. Adding one methyl group to amphetamine makes the drug much more potent. Adolescent use has remained stable or has declined over the years. The average elimination half-life of methamphetamine (12 hours) is much longer than that of cocaine (1 hour). Smoking crystal methamphetamine (ice, crystal, speed, tweak, crank, glass) can produce a high that lasts 8–24 hours. Besides euphoria, it increases wakefulness, increases the sexual drive, decreases appetite, and increases self-confidence. Use leads to depletion of the neurotransmitters, and users "crash" as the drug metabolizes, leaving them feeling depressed, somnolent, and hungry. These feelings cause them to re-seek the positive rewards. It has been associated with severe dental caries, psychosis, stroke from hypertension, myocardial infarction, arrhythmias, and exposure to HIV and other STDs because of risky sexual behaviors. Hyperthermia and convulsions can cause death.

Methamphetamine is extremely addictive, with many users becoming addicted after only a few uses. Tolerance occurs quickly, necessitating increasing doses, and it is relatively inexpensive and readily available! It causes neural "damage" from marked increase in dopamine in the synapse [Hanson, Rau *et al.*, 2004]. Chronic use depletes neurotransmitters and leads to chronic depression, requiring more of the drug to feel normal. The most important part of methamphetamine treatment is prevention. All adolescents must be repeatedly counseled to not try this drug even once. The regular user must not only be treated with drug abuse counseling, but in many instances, require an inpatient treatment program and intensive follow-up.

Acute Reactions to Drugs of Abuse

Cocaine can be swallowed, "snorted", or injected intravenously. It can be converted to the base as a residue (freebase) or solid (crack) that can be smoked. The duration of cocaine toxicity is usually brief because the drug has an elimination half-life of 1 hour. Cardiovascular toxicity includes sinus tachycardia, supraventricular or ventricular arrhythmias, and severe hypertension that may lead to cerebral hemorrhage. Myocardial infarction has been reported in patients with and without pre-existing coronary artery disease. Central nervous system (CNS) effects of cocaine include anxiety, agitation, paranoia, delirium, seizures, cerebral vasculitis and strokes. Hyperthermia can occur.

Heroin is usually injected intravenously but the powder can be "snorted" or smoked. Heroin overdose leads to respiratory depression, pulmonary edema, coma, bradycardia and hypotension. The acute toxic effects of other narcotics are generally similar to those of heroin, but may persist for up to several days with long-acting opioids such as methadone. A dose of 2 mg of naloxone (Narcan) intravenously will reverse the toxicity of most opioids; if necessary, the dose can be repeated at 2- to 3-minute intervals up to a total of 10 mg. Administration of naloxone to opioid-dependent patients can precipitate acute opioid withdrawal with severe agitation, as well as anxiety, piloerection, yawning, sneezing, rhinorrhea, nausea, vomiting, diarrhea and abdominal or muscle cramps.

The principal toxic effects of *sedative-hypnotics* are respiratory depression and coma, which may require endotracheal intubation and assisted ventilation. Many sedative-hypnotics, particularly in combination with other drugs, may also cause hypotension. Oral benzodiazepines alone are rarely lethal, but they are dangerous when taken with alcohol or other CNS depressants. Excessive alcohol ingestion, particularly in adolescents, may cause hypoglycemia; obtunded patients with possible alcohol ingestion should receive intravenous glucose.

Use of nitrous oxide or volatile *inhalants* such as gasoline, propane, freon or others can cause ataxia, respiratory depression and coma; some of these agents can also cause hepatic, renal or cardiac toxicity. Toluene (found in paint and glue) can cause hypokalemia, hypophosphatemia, renal tubular acidosis, abdominal pain, respiratory failure, and permanent neurologic deficits including ataxia. Sudden death following hydrocarbon inhalation is presumably due to cardiac arrhythmias.

Phencyclidine (PCP, Angel Dust) overdose can last for days and may cause psychosis or violent behavior. Severe overdose may cause coma, seizures, hypo- or hypertension, and muscular rigidity accompanied by severe hyperthermia and rhabdomyolysis.

Hallucinogens such as LSD or mescaline produce a hyper-suggestible state. Large doses of MDMA ("ecstasy"), MDA and other "designer" drugs similar in structure may produce amphetamine-like stimulant effects such as hyperthermia, hyponatremia and cerebral infarction, in addition to perceptual and behavioral effects.

Marijuana, hashish and *cannibinol* compounds can cause acute dysphoric reactions, sometimes associated with tachycardia and orthostatic hypotension. Usually, no specific treatment is needed, but severe reactions may respond to benzodiazepines.

Anabolic or androgenic steroids abused by athletes to enhance strength can cause aggressiveness, irritability, impaired judgment, impulsiveness, mania and paranoid delusions. Compulsive use and withdrawal symptoms have been reported.

Illicitly manufactured drugs may contain contaminants, toxic impurities and adulterants. Bacterial or fungal contaminants in intravenous (IV) drugs can cause sepsis or endocarditis, and the incidence of HIV infection is high among IV drug abusers. Talc in tablets which are crushed and then injected intravenously may cause pulmonary granulomas.

Diagnosis and Treatment of Substance Abuse Disorder

Comprehensive evaluation for substance abuse disorder is needed when there is continued use of a drug or alcohol in the presence of harmful consequences, such as continued use of marijuana with failing grades, legal problems, or family disapproval. Some adolescents may present as known regular drug users, but there is the rare circumstance when a patient admits to regular use and wants help. Assessment of severity of drug use will determine the level of treatment needed, and often diagnosis and management of a substance abuse disorder is best made by referral to a specialist in addiction medicine. Adolescents who regularly use drugs or alcohol often require a major intervention. A primary care clinician may be involved in monitoring urine drug screens in follow-up after treatment.

Diagnosis of Substance Use *Disorder* Requires Significant Impairment or Distress, with at least three of the following within a year

1. Tolerance: suggests physiologic dependence; a need for markedly increased amounts of the substance to achieve intoxication or desired effect, or diminished effect with continued use of the same amount of the substance.
2. Withdrawal: suggests physiologic dependence; characteristic withdrawal syndrome for the substance or a substance is taken to relieve or avoid withdrawal symptoms.
3. Substance is taken in larger amounts or over a longer period than was intended; suggests physiologic dependence.
4. There is a persistent desire or unsuccessful efforts to cut down or control substance use.

5. Much time is spent trying to obtain the substance (e.g. visiting many doctors or driving long distances), using the substance (e.g. chain-smoking), or recovering from its effects.
6. Important social, occupational, or recreational activities are given up or reduced because of use.
7. The substance use is continued in spite of knowledge of having a persistent or recurrent physical or psychological problem that is probably caused or made worse by the drug (e.g. current cocaine use despite recognition of cocaine-induced depression, or continued drinking despite recognition that an ulcer occurred from alcohol use).

Diagnosis of *Dependence* or *Abuse* is Recurrent Use Causing Impairment or Distress, with any continued use

- resulting in failed responsibilities at work, school, or home (e.g. repeated absences or poor work performance related to substance use; substance-related absences, suspensions, or expulsions from school; neglect of children or household).
- in situations in which it is physically hazardous (e.g. driving an automobile or operating a machine when impaired by the substance).
- with associated legal problems (e.g. arrests for substance-related disorderly conduct).
- despite having persistent or recurrent social or interpersonal problems caused or exacerbated by the effects of the substance (e.g. arguments with parents or partners about consequences of intoxication, physical fights).

Adolescents with substance abuse disorders need to be treated first for substance abuse, even if the substance use developed as an attempt to self-medicate mood or anxiety symptoms. Although substance abuse may cause mood and anxiety symptoms, or they may have developed as a way to cope with stress or symptoms, the substance use disorder must be treated before, or along with, any mood or anxiety disorder. Suicidal thinking must always be evaluated at both initial and follow-up visits for all adolescents with substance abuse.

Testing Adolescents for Substances of Abuse

Requests by parents, guardians or schools for laboratory testing for the presence of substances of abuse in minors should be referred early to an adolescent specialist or psychology personnel (rather than simply ordering a laboratory test) because of the extended time involved in comprehensive evaluation. A parental complaint of possible drug use is often a symptom of other personal or family problems requiring comprehensive evaluation. Drug testing of adolescents without a firm family and patient commitment to counseling or treatment may be counterproductive in terms of follow-up or changing drug-use behavior. Drug screening by a clinician without a family and patient commitment to an evaluation or a treatment program may further alienate or polarize the involved adolescent from supportive family or counseling resources. Since laboratory screening tests have inherent inaccuracies (30% in some studies and false negatives common after 2–3 days), they must be interpreted within the context of a comprehensive evaluation. Alcohol (abuse not readily detectable by drug testing) is the drug most frequently abused by teenagers and most commonly involved in teen drug-related deaths.

A 14-year-old male was brought to the clinician for a drug test by his mother who stated that he was always acting angry, and failing school. The patient completed a screening questionnaire (see pages 12–13) while the mother was interviewed in another room; she had told him he was going to the doctor for a "checkup to see what is wrong with him". The patient lives together with the mother, father (a night worker), and a younger sister. The mother reported that the patient stays up late at night, locked in his bedroom. He is often truant or late for school, and often comes home after dinner, when the father is at work. The patient admitted to her that he "tried" marijuana in the past, but he sometimes smells like smoke. She knew many of his friends about a year ago, but knows few now. She has searched his bedroom and found nothing drug-related.

The patient was then interviewed alone and his questionnaire responses were reviewed with him:

1. In the last 6 months, have you driven or been in a car when the driver was drinking or on drugs? Yes
2. Are you now taking any medicines, birth control pills, or other drugs? No
3. Do you ever drink alcohol, smoke, or take other drugs (besides medications prescribed for you)? Yes
4. Would you like birth control information or pamphlets? No
5. Are you having problems at home, at school, or with friends? Yes
6. Do you currently have a male and/or female lover? (If "Yes," circle which one) No
7. In the past 2 weeks have you felt down, depressed or hopeless? No
8. Have you ever had genital sexual contact (including vaginal, anal or oral sex)? No

9. Have you ever seriously thought about killing yourself, made a plan, or actually tried to kill yourself? No
10. In the last month, did you ride in a vehicle without a seatbelt on? Yes
11. Is there anything else you would like to discuss with the doctor or health provider? No

The patient stated that he rode home in the car with his father a few months ago when the father had a few beers, and rarely wears a seatbelt. He said that he smokes about five cigarettes a day, and that his mother probably knows that. When asked the *last* time he had marijuana, he said he could not remember. Upon review of the calendar, and with the understanding that a drug test will detect it for about a month, he confirmed that he "probably tried" it 3 weeks ago. He denied taking any other drugs or pills, or ever trying ice (meth), but he did say that he sniffed glue 4 months ago, and got drunk last month with friends. Most of his friends "smoke and drink sometimes." He described school as boring, and had no particular career interest or hobbies. He said his father is a dictator, and said his mother is always nagging him. He stays up late at night chatting online with friends or playing Internet games, and virtually never does homework. When asked if he had any ideas how to help his mother with her concerns about his schoolwork, smoking and disagreements, he recommended she just stop nagging him. Presented with the assumption that she expects him to succeed in school and not use drugs or marijuana, he stated he can agree to attend school and stay clean from marijuana. It was proposed to him that we inform his mother together that his marijuana drug test would be positive today and that he agrees not to smoke it further, expecting tests to remain negative beginning in a week. He agreed to see a "counselor" to get him back on track in school and to learn ways to "handle his family." While he read some information, the mother was *separately* counseled that he would benefit from counseling for a variety of issues, and that he is willing to stay clean from drugs, although a test today would be positive for marijuana, making it unnecessary to order and pay for one. Then, *together*, the situation was reviewed as described above, and the patient was informed that the mother can have him tested at her discretion beginning in a week. They agreed to a referral to a male social worker counselor experienced in substance abuse and family therapy, and the father will be encouraged to attend. The school counselor will arrange a tracking system for his attendance and homework. He will return for follow-up in 2 weeks, then as needed.

Clinical Issues

There are unanswered questions regarding informed consent and physician-patient confidentiality in drug screening of minors at a parent's insistence. A clinician ordering such a test without the minor's consent or without a comprehensive consultation may be at risk for not meeting standards of care, and the clinician should explain to the parent the need for proper referral to an adolescent specialist, chemical dependency specialist, or psychology personnel. There are also concerns about proper interpretation of test results, their real meaning, and who is to be informed of results, as well as handling and confidentiality of medical records. Often, there are cost issues since drug screening may not be covered by a health plan unless medically necessary (i.e. acute overdose requiring treatment). The cost and inclusiveness of the laboratory test varies depending on the number of substances included in the ordered test.

Urine drug screens are often indicated when an adolescent is already in outpatient drug treatment and has consented to ongoing monitoring; these may be performed regularly or randomly with visual observation of the collection of the specimen. Other circumstances for testing may include: being caught at school with drugs, needing testing for employment, and the desire of a patient for a test to prove he or she is drug free.

It is necessary to inform the parent of a minor that a lab test only measures possible drug use and that the sensitivity of a typical urine test is 2–4 weeks for marijuana and 2–4 days for many other drugs. False negatives are common and many are only detectable for a short time after use, and may not be found at the time a teen is tested. A negative drug test does not rule out a substance abuse problem since certain tests may not detect all illicit drugs used by teens. It is possible for a patient to create a negative drug test by drinking excessive water or using products from nutritional supplement stores. "False-positive" results may occur for some drugs that remain detectable for a while after a teen has quit using. Many prescription medications, antibiotics, some common over-the-counter painkillers, decongestants, allergy medications or even foods can be misinterpreted by a test as an illicit drug; a teen under parents' suspicion may particularly resent this kind of result.

A positive drug test result in a medical chart may affect future health insurability, life insurance applications and government security clearances, etc. Home test kits often give false or deceptive results. Accurate or not, those tests can create bad feelings where a teen resents parental distrust and becomes even less open. A resentful teen is less likely to turn to parents for support that helps deter drug use.

A Clinical Approach

Interview the parent first, while the teen is completing a written questionnaire or comprehensive computerized screening. Simple written questions may include (from pages 12–13):

- In the last 6 months, have you driven or been in a car when the driver was drinking or on drugs?
- Are you now taking any medicines, birth control pills, or other drugs?
- Do you ever drink alcohol, smoke, or take other drugs (besides medications prescribed for you)?
- Are you having problems at home, at school, or with friends?

Comprehensive computerized screening by the Youth Health Program (see Appendix) allows presetting the Question Mode to a specialized Drug Screening assessment for an evaluation.

Screening Interview of the Parent
- Does the teen know why he or she is here? What was he or she told?
- Who does the teen live with? Family problems/issues?
- Explore situation or problem behaviors.
- Explore trend in school grades and behaviors.
- Past known drug use?
- Was the teen seen or found intoxicated?
- Any money, valuables or alcohol missing?
- Did anybody report known drug use by the teen?
- Has the teen been found with any drugs or paraphernalia?
- The teen's friends' characteristics and any known drug use.

Ask the parents to remain separate from the adolescent during interview of the adolescent, but assure the parents that they will be included later. It is optimal to obtain a drug use history by referring to answers to the screening questions, after informing the adolescent that certain substances may appear in a urine test for about a month.

Screening interview of the patient (without a parent present, after the review of the screening questionnaire)

- What is your parent concerned about? What's going on?
- Any marijuana use within the past 30 days?
- Any ice/speed/amphetamines use ever?

- When was the last time you had any drugs, and which one(s)?
- Any drinking of alcohol on weekends or on weekdays? Quantity each time?

It may be useful to look at a calendar together with the adolescent and ask him or her to show the last use date, indicating that "a drug test can detect drugs for a month or more." If the patient admits to drug use within 4 weeks for marijuana or 4 days for other drugs, then inform the patient that it may be better to admit to the use rather than have a positive test occur. Ask the teen if and how he or she would like to inform the parents, and reassure the teen that the clinician will support the idea of obtaining a future result to prove no further drug use. Ask the patient if he or she can commit to staying off drugs and guarantee negative future tests.

Meet with the parent and teen together; explain that the test is "positive" by interview, and that it is optimal to obtain a negative laboratory test after the date when we would expect the drug to clear (i.e. 4 weeks after marijuana use). When appropriate, in front of the teen, provide the parent with the ability to take their teen to be tested at their discretion. Consent for any testing must be obtained from the minor, and any forced testing can damage the relationship between a teen and a physician.

Ethical Issues

It is not ethical to order a test if the minor refuses; involuntary or surreptitious drug testing, in particular, may undermine a teen's trust in health providers. Even results that show no drug use can be harmful if a teen feels coerced into the test. Most teens can stop using drugs with their parents' care, concern and supervision, as well as a personal desire to change their lives. Many youths stop misusing alcohol or drugs as they reach late adolescence. However, some adolescents do need specialized help to quit, such as individual or group counseling, or even residential treatment in the case of serious substance abuse.

Drug testing athletes in secondary schools can be an incentive to not participate in extracurricular athletic activities; they can be discouraged from participating in the very activities that can have a positive impact on their lives. Extracurricular activities are a form of prevention (and even treatment) for drug abuse — not as a privilege to be revoked from drug-abusing students. It is estimated that 5% of schools in America drug-test their student athletes, and it is most common in rural school districts. Unfortunately, students can have such personal medical information become common knowledge. Most medical societies do not support routine drug screening. The testing of adolescent *professional* athletes for anabolic steroids is rarely the clinician's domain.

Involuntary drug testing is advisable only in an emergency or if the adolescent lacks decision making capacity. Clinicians should advise parents about the limitations and potential risks associated with home drug-testing products as well as the inaccuracies of Internet-based recommendations intended for parents. There is little consistency among physicians about how to proceed when a drug test is positive, but testing is best used as part of a drug treatment program.

Attention Deficit Disorder

Attention Deficit Disorder (ADD) is a common behavioral disorder of childhood and adolescence [Yiming, 2008]. Common symptoms for making the diagnosis in childhood are persistent inattention and distractibility, and sometimes, hyperactivity and/or impulsivity with Attention-Deficit-Hyperactivity Disorder (ADHD). It is difficult to initially diagnose during adolescence since the diagnosis is almost always made by 11 years of age. Research shows that ADHD is a common familial-genetic condition, with inheritability found 80% of the time. In some countries, ADHD is diagnosed in 1 out of 10 children. When accurately diagnosed during childhood, it persists into adolescence in 80% of those children, leaving about 8% of all adolescents with ADHD, mostly males.

Diagnostic Criteria Required for Attention Deficit Disorder Both With and Without Hyperactivity
- Some inattentive, distractive, hyperactive, or impulsive symptoms were present before age 11.
- Current impairment in social, academic, or vocational areas.
- Current symptoms are not part of another developmental or mental disorder, and have persisted for 6 months or more.

Diagnostic Criteria for Attention Deficit Disorder Without Hyperactivity
- Cannot pay adequate attention to schoolwork, work, or other activities, with difficulty sustaining attention in tasks.
- Does not listen effectively when spoken to or understand instructions adequately.
- Does not finish schoolwork or duties in the workplace.
- Has difficulty organizing tasks and activities.
- Avoids or dislikes tasks that require continual mental focus (e.g. schoolwork, homework).
- Is easily distracted by extraneous stimuli.
- Often forgetful in daily activities.

Diagnostic Criteria for Attention Deficit Disorder with Hyperactivity

- Fidgety or squirms while seated.
- Leaves or gets up from seat in classroom or in other situations when being seated is normal.
- Moves around or feels restless.
- Has difficulty in quiet leisure activities.
- Speaks before others are done speaking.
- Finds it hard to wait for a turn.
- Interrupts or intrudes on others.
- Is accident prone.

Some symptoms can occur in adolescents who are bored with work or subjects being addressed. Diagnosis of ADD in adolescents is complicated by normal fluctuations in mood and other conditions such as substance abuse. Teacher rating scales of behaviors (e.g. Vanderbilt, Conners) are difficult to apply to adolescents, and it is common for secondary school students to have numerous teachers who are only with them a few hours a week. When feasible, feedback from as many teachers as possible can help in the assessment of the adolescent with possible ADD. The assessment of the adolescent also should include a complete history and physical examination (including family history for ADD), and a mental status evaluation including screening for depression. School records and academic testing should be reviewed, and the possibility of an unrecognized, specific learning disability or other intellectual disability should be ruled out [Peat, Tan, 2008].

Management

Management may include stimulant medication, but a positive response to stimulant medication does not confirm the diagnosis of ADD, since adolescents without ADD can have improved attention and performance with stimulant medication. A brief trial of coffee (caffeine) at breakfast and lunch may prove useful if the adolescent can subjectively describe positive responses to this preliminary evaluation. It is often necessary to enlist the adolescent patient to assist (documenting both subjectively and objectively) during any diagnostic trials of medications. Begin medication at a low dose and increase it until symptoms improve and are acceptable to the adolescent, parents, and teachers. Ritalin and amphetamine are first choice medications for most adolescents with ADHD. Careful titration of stimulants offers best treatment outcomes.

Other therapies used for adolescents with ADHD include:

1. Psychotherapy to help develop strategies to optimize performance.
2. Cognitive-behavior therapy to help youths make appropriate behavior changes by changing thoughts and feelings.

3. Brainwave biofeedback to create brain-based functional change and ability to relax and control responses to stressors.
4. Psychosocial treatments that include social skills training, support groups, and parent-teacher training.
6. Classroom behavior modification, academic interventions, and special education placement.

Nearly All Adolescents with ADHD Have a Comorbid Condition; two-thirds have two or more of these:

- Oppositional defiant disorder.
- Conduct disorder.
- Mood or anxiety disorder: Adolescents with ADHD are often upset or depressed due to their problems, which result in low self-esteem. Most adolescents with ADHD have a mood disorder, and those with bipolar disorder are difficult to treat.
- Learning disability: Some adolescents have a specific information processing deficit. About a quarter of children with ADHD have a specific learning disability.
- Academic achievement problem: Above-average intellectual ability and below-average academic achievement is common. Most adolescents with ADD do not have specific learning disabilities, but have academic achievement problems, with more school dropout.
- Substance abuse: Adolescents with ADD use more cigarettes, alcohol and marijuana (mostly in those with conduct disorder).
- Family relation problems: Adolescents with ADHD have more negative interactions, more family conflict and underestimate the amount of conflict when compared to their parents.
- High-risk sexual behaviors: Adolescents with ADHD have an earlier age of first sexual intercourse, more sexual partners, less use of birth control, more sexually transmitted diseases, and more teen pregnancies.

Other Psychological and Behavioral Issues for Adolescents

There are many other psychological and behavioral issues that impact on the lives of adolescents, but three of them remain a particular concern for parents and clinicians.

Media Exposure

The alcohol industry, with impunity and without restraint, advertises in magazines and TV programs that have primarily young audiences. This advertising has significant impact on youths. Similarly, brand advertising not only sells cigarettes, but also sells the social acceptability of smoking. Advertisements make smoking seem exciting, glamorous, and even healthy.

Many adolescents worldwide are exposed to violent media, and the primary care clinician *can* impact this problem. Counseling about television and other media with parents of children can yield results later. Many scientific studies show that children learn violent attitudes and behavior from watching violence on television, particularly those already prone to aggression. Half of American television programs (distributed worldwide) contain some violence. There is a proven association of media violence to aggressive behavior, and media violence is estimated to cause about a fifth of real-life violence. The clinician should counsel against exposure to violent media (especially first-person shooter video games and violent movies) at young ages.

Basic Media Guidelines for Parents

- Limit recreational TV and Internet to 2 hours a day.
- Do not use TV or Internet as a reward or punishment (increases importance).
- Encourage parent-child co-viewing.
- Monitor programs watched, and minimize violence exposure.
- Use lockout devices to limit viewing of restricted material.
- Offer alternative entertainment options.
- Discuss programs viewed, particularly reality vs fiction.
- Teach resistance to TV commercials, and regularly mute their sound.

Internet Risks

The Internet is already in the lives of most adolescents worldwide. It has created a digital media culture in the new millennium. The most popular use of the Internet is for communication, such as e-mail, interactive games, instant messaging with friends, and real-time chatting. Large numbers of adolescents use the Internet to access health information in an anonymous and non-judgmental way. Adolescents need to know that not all information placed on the Internet is accurate or true. There are some associated risks, as with all media, and many other activities. Some reports indicate that 1 in 5 teens receive an unwanted sexual solicitation annually on the Internet, but few lead to an actual sexual contact or assault. Online relationships are an uncharted area of psychological research; relationship development online differs from that offline. Wolak [2003] reported that 1 in 7 youths had close online friendships during the past year. Of these online Internet relationships, 70% were with same-age peers, 71% crossed gender lines, 74% were known to parents (a third were initiated by friends or family), 70% had offline contact by mail or telephone, 41% had face-to-face meetings, and 12% reported online romances.

There have been studies suggesting psychological harm from too much time spent on the Internet, but other studies have not shown a causal relationship between Internet use and psychological problems. Information overload is an issue, but serious problems are the exception and are non-specific. The Internet does not create new pathologies, and excessive use and isolation (most common with male adolescents) should be solved on an educational basis. The Internet can be a practical, effective and efficient way to deliver health information to adolescents (see Chapter 9). Clinicians and parents should be proactive in defining Internet quality, and understand how technology will facilitate, amplify, and alter the cognitive processes and social behavior of the Internet generation.

Internet Safety for Adolescents
- Do not give out identifying information.
- Ignore obscene, threatening messages.
- Meetings require parental permission.
- Limit recreational time (as with TV and telephone).
- Parents should know where their children go online.
- Parents should make ground rules, and the teen should sign a contract.

Adolescent Drivers

Automobile crashes are the leading cause of death among adolescent males. One of the most dangerous driving maneuvers for adolescents is making left turns. In some studies, when compared to adults, adolescent drivers detected the appearance of the cross-traffic cars significantly more slowly in test videos, and allowed cars to get significantly closer compared to middle-aged drivers. Consistent with statistics, adolescents have more violations and crashes than middle-aged drivers. This may be partly due to adolescents taking longer to detect a driving stimulus such as a car appearing on the horizon [Cox, 2001]. Adolescents with ADHD have even poorer driving skills, more accidents and traffic citations, especially those with oppositional defiant disorder or conduct disorder.

A *Contract for a Teen Driver* is highly recommended for beginning adolescent drivers. Parental conditions and restrictions may include a Graduated Drivers License privilege, with restrictions on passengers and driving between 7 p.m. and 6 a.m. It should also include an adolescent's promise not to get into a car where the driver has consumed alcohol or drugs, and a parent's promise to pick him or her up without questions (or pay for a taxi to come home) if the adolescent is ever intoxicated.

Contract for a Teen Driver

Teen Driver

I promise not to get into a car where the driver has consumed alcohol or drugs.

I promise not to drive under the influence of alcohol or drugs.

If I am ever in need of a ride home for my safety, I will ask for a designated driver, call a taxi or call a parent or another family member for a ride. I will always find an alternate means home if I am ever in a situation where the driver has been drinking or using drugs.

I promise to wear my seatbelt when driving or riding in a car (in both the front and back seat). I will not eat or listen to loud music while driving, and my cell phone will be turned off or silenced.

I will get permission in advance to use the car, as well as let a parent know my whereabouts with the car at all times. I will never let another person drive the car, or drive a car I am not insured for — even with the owner's permission.

I will pay the added cost of insurance with accidents or moving violations.

Signature of Teen Driver

Parent(s)/Guardian(s)

I promise to pick you up if you ever call me for a ride because you are not safe to drive. If that is not possible, I will pay for a taxi to bring you home.

I also promise not to start a conversation about the incident at that time.

I will not drive under the influence of drugs or alcohol, and will find an alternate means home if I am ever in a situation where the driver has been drinking or using drugs.

Signatures of Parent(s)/Guardian(s)

Suggested Readings and Bibliography

Abramowicz M (ed). (1996). Acute reactions to drugs of abuse. *Med Lett Drugs Ther*, 38, pp. 43–46.

American Academy of Pediatrics, Committee on Adolescence. (2000). Suicide and suicide attempts in adolescents. *Pediatrics*, 105, pp. 871–874.

American Academy of Pediatrics, Committee on Child Abuse and Neglect. (1999). Guidelines for the evaluation of sexual abuse of children: subject review. *Pediatrics*, 103, pp. 186–191.

American Academy of Pediatrics, Committee on Substance Abuse. (1998). Tobacco, alcohol, and other drugs: the role of the pediatrician in prevention and management of substance abuse. *Pediatrics*, 101, pp. 125–128.

American Academy of Pediatrics, Committee on Substance Abuse; American Academy of Pediatrics, Council on School Health, Knight JR, *et al.* (2007). Testing for drugs of abuse in children and adolescents: addendum — testing in schools and at home. *Pediatrics*, 119, pp. 627–630.

American Academy of Pediatrics, Committee on Substance Abuse. (2001). Alcohol use and abuse: a pediatric concern. *Pediatrics*, 108, pp. 185–189.

American Psychiatric Association. (1994). *Diagnostic and Statistical Manual of Mental Disorders (DSM-IV)*. 4th Edn. (American Psychiatric Association, Washington).

Atabaki S, Paradise JE. (1999). The medical evaluation of the sexually abused child. *Pediatrics*, 104, pp. 178–186.

Berdie J, Baizerman M, Lourie I. (1977). Violence towards youth: themes from a workshop. *Children Today*, 6, pp. 7–10, 35.

Brent DA, Birmaher B. (2002). Cinical practice. Adolescent depression. *N Engl J Med*, 347, pp. 667–671.

Beck AT, Steer RA, Brown GK. (1987). *Beck Depression Inventory*. (Psychological Corporation, San Antonio).

Barangan CJ, Alderman EM. (2002). Management of substance abuse. *Pediatr Rev*, 23, pp. 123–131.

Belson WA. (1978). *Television Violence and the Adolescent Boy*. (Saxon House, Westmead).

Borzekowski DL. (2006). Adolescents' use of the Internet: a controversial, coming-of-age resource. *Adolesc Med Clin*, 17, pp. 205–216.

Carlson GA, Cantwell DP. (1980). Unmasking masked depression in children and adolescents. *Am J Psychiatry*, 137, pp. 445–449.

Cheung AH, Zuckerbrot RA, Jensen PS, Ghalib K, Laraque D, Stein RE; GLAD-PC Steering Group. (2007). Guidelines for Adolescent Depression in Primary Care (GLAD-PC): II. Treatment and ongoing management. *Pediatrics*, 120, pp. e1313–1326. (Erratum in: *Pediatrics*, 121, p. 227).

Clarke GN, Rohde P, Lewinsohn PM, Hops H, Seeley JR. (1999). Cognitive-behavioral treatment of adolescent depression: efficacy of acute group treatment and booster sessions. *J Am Acad Child Adolesc Psychiatry*, 38, pp. 272–279.

Coyle JT, Pine DS, Charney DS, *et al.* (2003). Depression and bipolar support alliance consensus statement on the unmet needs in diagnosis and treatment of mood disorders in children and adolescents. *J Am Acad Child Adolesc Psychiatry*, 42, pp. 1494–1503.

Cox B, Cox D, Tuite M. (2001). Driving difficulties among male adolescents. *J Adolesc Health*, 29, pp. 312–313.

Deisher R, Eisner V, Sulzbacher S. (1969). The young male prostitute. *Pediatrics*, 43, pp. 936–941.

Deisher RW, Wenet GA, Paperny DM, *et al.* (1982). Adolescent sexual offense behavior: the role of the physician. *J Adolescent Health Care*, 2, pp. 279–286.

Deisher RW. (1975). Runaways: a growing social and family problem. *J Fam Pract*, 2, pp. 255–258.

Eisenberg ME, Aalsma MC; Society for Adolescent Medicine. (2005). Bullying and peer victimization: position paper of the Society for Adolescent Medicine. *J Adolesc Health*, 36, pp. 88–91.

Evans DL, Foa EB, Gur RE, *et al.* (eds). (2005). *Treating and Preventing Adolescent Mental Health Disorders: What We Know and What We Don't Know*. (Oxford University Press, New York).

Ewing JA. (1984). Detecting alcoholism. The CAGE questionnaire. *JAMA*, 252, pp. 1905–1907.

Faber A, Mazlish E. (1980). *How To Talk So Kids Will Listen & Listen So Kids Will Talk.* (Avon Books, USA).

Fergusson DM, Woodward LJ, Horwood LJ. (2000). Risk factors and life processes associated with the onset of suicidal behavior during adolescence and early adulthood. *Psychol Med*, 30, pp. 23–39.

Fingerhur LA, Kleinman JC. (1990). International and interstate comparisons of homicide among young males. *JAMA*, 263, pp. 3292–3294.

Garrett BL, Silver MP. (1976). The use of EMG and alpha biofeedback to relieve test anxiety in college students. In: I. Wickramasekera (Ed), *Biofeedback, Behavior Therapy, and Hypnosis.* (Nelson-Hall, Chicago).

Gilbody S, Whitty P, Grimshaw J, Thomas R. (2003). Educational and organizational interventions to improve the management of depression in primary care: a systematic review. *JAMA*, 289, pp. 3145–3151.

Green WH. (2001). *Child and Adolescent Psychopharmacology.* (Lippincott, Williams and Wilkins, Baltimore).

Grunbaum JA, Kann L, Kinchen S, *et al.* (2004). Youth Risk Behavior Surveillance–United States, 2003 (Abridged). *J Sch Health*, 74, pp. 307–324.

Gushurst C, Palusci V. (2010). Medical evaluation of child sexual abuse. In: Greydanus D, Patel D, Reddy V, Feinberg A, Omar H (eds), *Handbook of Clinical Pediatrics: An Update for the Ambulatory Pediatrician*, pp. 668–693. (World Scientific Publishing, Singapore).

Hammond DC. (2001). Neurofeedback treatment of depression with the Roshi. *Journal of Neurotherapy*, 4, pp. 45–56.

Hanson GR, Rau KS, Fleckenstein AE. (2004). The methamphetamine experience: a NIDA partnership. *Neuropharmacology*, 47 (Suppl 1), pp. 92–100.

Kaul P, Coupey SM. (2002). Clinical evaluation of substance abuse. *Pediatr Rev* 23, pp. 85–93.

Levy S, Harris S, Sherritt L, *et al.* (2006). Drug testing of adolescents in general medical clinics, in school and at home: physician attitudes and practices. *J Adolesc Health*, 38, pp. 336–342.

Lourie I. (1977). The phenomenon of the abused adolescent: A clinical study. *Victimology*, 2, pp. 268–276.

Levy S, Van Hook S, Knight J. (2004). A review of Internet-based home drug testing products for parents. *Pediatrics*, 113, pp. 720–726.

Lewinsohn PM, Essau CA. (2002). Depression in adolescents. In: Gotlib IH, Hammen CL (eds), *Handbook of Depression.* 8th Edn. pp. 541–559. (Guilford Press, New York).

Lubar JO, Lubar JF. (1984). Electroencephalographic biofeedback of SMR and beta for treatment of attention deficit disorders in a clinical setting. *Biofeedback Self Regul*, 9, pp. 1–23.

Maguire J, Philadelphia Child Guidance Center, Philip Lief Group. (1995). *Your Child's Emotional Health: Adolescence.* (Macmillan, USA).

Moore NC. (2000). A review of EEG biofeedback treatment of anxiety disorders. *Clin Electroencephalogr*, 31, pp. 1–6.

Mufson L, Dorta KP, Wickramaratne P, Nomura Y, Olfson M, Weissman MM. (2004). A randomized effectiveness trial of interpersonal psychotherapy for depressed adolescents. *Arch Gen Psychiatry*, 61, pp. 577–584.

Olfson M, Shaffer D, Marcus SC, *et al.* (2003). Relationship between antidepressant medication treatment and suicide in adolescents. *Arch Gen Psychiatry*, 60, pp. 978–982.

Othmer S, Othmer SF, Marks CS. (1991). EEG Biofeedback Training for Attention Deficit Disorder, Specific Learning Disabilities, and Associated Conduct Problems. Available from: http://www.eegspectrum.com/Applications/ADHD-ADD/ADD-SLD-ACPIntro.

Paperny D, Hicks R, Hammar SL. (1980). Munchausen's syndrome. *Am J Dis Child*, 134, pp. 794–795.

Paperny DH, Aono JY, Lehman RM, Hammar SL. (1988). Computer-assisted detection, evaluation, and referral of sexually abused adolescents. *J Adolesc Health Care*, 9, p. 260.

Paperny D, Deisher R. (1983). Maltreatment of adolescents: the relationship to a predisposition toward violent behavior and delinquency. *Adolescence*, 18, pp. 499–506.

Peat D, Tan E. (2008). Learing disorders. In: Fung D, Yiming C (eds), *A Primer of Child and Adolescent Psychiatry*, pp. 95–113. (World Scientific Publishing, Singapore).

Petchers MK, Singer MI. (1987). Perceived-Benefit-of-Drinking Scale: approach to screening for adolescent alcohol abuse. *J Pediatr*, 110, pp. 977–981.

Poirier MP. (2002). Care of the female adolescent rape victim. *Pediatr Emerg Care*, 18, pp. 53–59.

Reinherz, HZ, Giaconia, RM, Pakiz, B, *et al.* (1993). Psychosocial risks for major depression in late adolescence: a longitudinal community study. *J Am Acad Child Adolesc Psychiatry*, 32, p. 1155.

Reynolds WM, Lutz FL. (1987). Reynolds Adolescent Depression Scale. (Psychological Assessment Resources, Odessa).

Rosenberg D, *et al.* (1998). *Pocket Guide for the Textbook of Child and Adolescent Psychiatric Disorders*. (Taylor & Francis, Washington DC).

Rosenfeld JP. (2000). An EEG biofeedback protocol for affective disorders. *Clin Electroencephalogr*, 31, pp. 7–12.

Rushton JL, Clark SJ, Freed GL. (2000). Pediatrician and family physician prescription of selective serotonin reuptake inhibitors. *Pediatrics*, 105, p. E82.

Sakai C, Paperny D, Mathews M, *et al.* (2001). Thought Field Therapy clinical applications: utilization in an HMO in behavioral medicine and behavioral health services. *J Clin Psychol*, 57, pp. 1215–1227.

Saluja G, Iachan R, Scheidt PC, *et al.* (2004). Prevalence of and risk factors for depressive symptoms among young adolescents. *Arch Pediatr Adolesc Med*, 158, p. 760.

Saxby E, Peniston EG. (1995). Alpha-theta brainwave neurofeedback training: an effective treatment for male and female alcoholics with depressive symptoms. *J Clin Psychol*, 51, pp. 685–693.

Scott W, Kaiser D. (1998). Augmenting chemical dependency treatment with neurofeedback training. *Journal of Neurotherapy*, 3, p. 66.

Sege R, Stringham P, Short S, Griffith J. (1999). Ten years after: examination of adolescent screening questions that predict future violence-related injury. *J Adolesc Health*, 24, pp. 395–402.

Strasburger VC. (1997). Children, adolescents and television. A call for physician action. *West J Med*, 166, pp. 353–354.

Song G. (2008). Substance abuse and dependence. In: Fung D, Yiming C (eds), *A Primer of Child and Adolescent Psychiatry*, pp. 163–183. (World Scientific Publishing, Singapore).

Syed TS. (2004). Help the adolescent patient quit smoking. *J Pediatr Adolesc Gynecol*, 17, pp. 357–361.

URSA (Urban and Rural Systems Associates). (1980). Adolescent abuse and neglect: intervention strategies. U.S. Department of Health and Human Services-National Center on Child Abuse and Neglect (The User Manual Series), July, 1980.

Wolak J. (2003). Escaping or connecting? Characteristics of youth who form close online relationships. *J Adolesc*, 26, pp. 105–119.

Woo B. (2008). Emotional disorder In: Fung D, Yiming C (eds), *A Primer of Child and Adolescent Psychiatry*, pp. 55–74. (World Scientific Publishing, Singapore).

Yiming C. (2008). Attention deficit hyperactivity disorder. In: Fung D, Yiming C (eds), *A Primer of Child and Adolescent Psychiatry*, pp. 115–126. (World Scientific Publishing, Singapore).

Yiming C. (2008). Evaluation of antisocial behaviors; conduct disorder. In: Fung D, Yiming C (eds), *A Primer of Child and Adolescent Psychiatry*, pp. 249–265. (World Scientific Publishing, Singapore).

Yiming C, Kee C. (2008). Adolescent smoking. In: Fung D, Yiming C (eds), *A Primer of Child and Adolescent Psychiatry*, pp. 185–191. (World Scientific Publishing, Singapore).

Zuckerbrot RA, Cheung AH, Jensen PS, Stein RE, Laraque D; GLAD-PC Steering Group. (2007). Guidelines for Adolescent Depression in Primary Care (GLAD-PC): I. Identification, assessment, and initial management. *Pediatrics*, 120, pp. e1299–1312.

Zuckerbrot RA, Maxon L, Pagar D, Davies M, Fisher PW, Shaffer D. (2007). Adolescent depression screening in primary care: feasibility and acceptability. *Pediatrics*, 119, pp. 101–108.

Suggested Websites

Resilience Net: http://resilnet.uiuc.edu

The Academy for Eating Disorders is a global professional association committed to leadership in eating disorders research, education, treatment, and prevention: http://www.aedweb.org

Children and Adults with Attention Deficit/Hyperactivity Disorder (CHADD) is a national non-profit organization for children and adults with attention-deficit/hyperactivity disorder and their families. This site contains fact sheets on the diagnosis and treatment of AD/HD, legal rights, parenting, and education, legislative information, organizational information, and an online store for ordering annual conference audio and video tapes, fact sheets in bulk, and books: http://www.chadd.org

National Clearinghouse for Alcohol and Drug Information is a service of the U.S. Substance Abuse and Mental Health Services Admin. This site provides a wide range of online resources on drugs and alcohol, including reports on the annual Household Survey on Drug Abuse, a database and web search engines, research information, online courses for professionals, publications for parents and teens, a kids' area, and related links: http://www.health.org or http://ncadi.samhsa.gov

National Institute on Drug Abuse: This site contains a wide range of reports and information (both professional and lay) on drugs of abuse including steroids, club drugs, and tobacco; research, and advisories, access to NIDA Notes (a bimonthly newsletter), NIDA InfoFax (fact sheets on drug abuse in both English and Spanish), teaching support materials for schools, and the latest Monitoring the Future Study report on adolescent substance use/abuse: http://www.nida.nih.gov

Tips 4 Teens (of the U.S. Centers for Disease Control): This site provides resources for adolescents and young adults about smoking and tobacco. There is information about the hazards of smoking, how to quit, messages from the U.S. Surgeon General's reports on smoking, a teen media contest, order forms for free posters and publications. Links to other related sites are of interest to parents and youth leaders as well as teens: http://www.cdc.gov/HealthyYouth/az/index.htm. Similar information, but from an adult point of view, can be found at: http://www.cdc.gov/nccdphp/osh/tobacco.htm

The American Academy of Child and Adolescent Psychiatry: http://www.aacap.org/ Announcements/ psychiatricmeds.htm

The American Psychiatric Association: http://www.psych.org

Chapter 7

Adolescent Sexuality and Reproductive Health

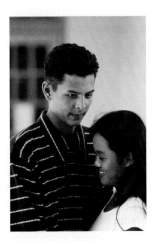

Adolescents around the world too often share a common experience: a lack of information about sexuality, little access to sexual health services, and the denial of their sexual and reproductive rights. Sexuality education [and learning Responsible Sexuality] is a life-long process of acquiring information and forming attitudes, beliefs, and values. It is unacceptable that adolescents throughout the world are still lacking the basic facts they need to make informed, [healthy] decisions about their sexual and reproductive lives.

— SIECUS.org

171

Overview

We are all sexual beings from cradle to grave. Sexuality is not a genie in a bottle which pops out at puberty. The quality of its expression changes over time with development. Sexuality is, however, one of the five major tasks of adolescence: to become comfortable with sexuality, and achieving maturity about one's own sexuality. Young people will need to develop the knowledge, attitudes, and skills required to become sexually responsible, healthy adults. As they grow and mature, they need access to accurate information about sexuality. Parents, educators, and clinicians need to support them and provide high quality educational opportunities. *Responsible sexuality* should be the mainstay of health education as children grow into adults. The clinician's role is promotion of healthy psychosexual adjustment, and preventing the negative health consequences of sexual behaviors. The ultimate goal of clinical management is to reduce social and intrapsychic conflict as well as to prevent and treat disease. During different periods of adolescence and for individuals with various types of conflicts, treatment strategies may require cooperative efforts of several professional workers with different training and skills. Certain behaviors with high medical, social, and personal morbidity are particularly relevant to the adolescent.

Adolescent Sexual Psychology

The healthiest environment for sexual growth is one that provides positive experiences and models from which the individual can learn. Difficulties which adolescents commonly face in attaining a sense of competence and freedom vital to a pleasurable and normal adult sexual life are complicated by Western society's ambivalence towards sexuality [Eisenberg, 1969]. Young people today face a peculiar dilemma. Reaching their period of greatest sexual vigor several years before stable coupling or marriage are possible, they frequently find the doors to societally-sanctioned sexual activity closed. Early adolescents may have a fear of the intensity of their sexuality and sexual instincts.

Adolescent sexual attitudes are impacted by societal change; there exists: mixed sexual messages, instability of family, decreased religiosity, changed female role, long period between fecundity and marriage, more acceptance of premarital sex for young adults, and less stigma attached to unwed pregnancy and same-sex relationships. Nearly all adolescents will become sexually active between age 13–24, so sexuality refers to a broader range of issues including physical changes and interpersonal relationships. These are affected by early teens being cognitively limited and concrete; they are now-oriented, cannot foresee consequences, and are egocentric experimenters. Though middle teens are more abstract and can be more futuristic, peer influences dominate and there is denial of risk in order to take risk. Medical considerations for most adolescents must include the startling lack of awareness and understanding among many of the variety of diseases transmitted by sexual contacts. Many adolescents, although sexually very experienced, usually know much less than we frequently assume. Their unawareness of their exposure to diseases, symptoms of these diseases, risks of pregnancy, and the need to have periodic medical screening illustrates this.

Adolescents may have maladaptive psychosexual attitudes such as: "I am abstinent; I only have oral sex and anal sex, so I am still a virgin." Other maladaptive psychological processes often dominate early and middle adolescent thinking about sexuality.

Sexually Maladaptive Cognitive Processes
- Ignorance: "I didn't think I was having sex often enough to get pregnant. I thought there was something wrong with me and I couldn't get pregnant. I didn't know I could get birth control. I didn't know where to get birth control. I thought I was too young to get pregnant. I thought withdrawal was good protection."
- Denial: "I only had sex once. Sex should be spontaneous. I just haven't gotten around to birth control. I was waiting for a closer relationship with my boyfriend."
- Fear: "I'm afraid of the side effects. I'm afraid my parents would find out. I'm afraid of the pelvic exam."
- Personal fables: "I know I won't get pregnant. My boyfriend is really fast. I know when I'm fertile."

The physician's role is to optimize health outcomes. Disapproval of sexual behavior is unprofessional. Disagreement with poor choices is appropriate and must be carefully shared. Counseling and brief health advice (especially scare tactics) rarely changes behavior. Only 5% to 20% of adults change their health behaviors with good brief negotiation. However, adolescents are in situations making emotional choices not always under volitional control. "Don't ask, don't tell" is inadequate health care. The physician is obligated to (immediately) refer adolescent patients that he or she is unable or unwilling to thoroughly treat. It is the clinician's responsibility to understand the consequences and implications of sexually transmitted diseases and early childbearing, and treat them as *preventable* medical conditions.

Sexual Health Services

Over half of adolescents between ages 12–18 years are (vaginally) sexually experienced; this increases with age. Therefore, abstinent adolescents should be counseled about availability of services when their status changes. About 80% of females will become pregnant within a year without the use of contraception. In the United States, about half of all teenage pregnancies occur within the first 6 months of sexual activity, since they usually wait over a year after first intercourse before seeking sexual health services. Reflexive referral of female teens for gynecologic visits (which often never occur) is no longer the standard of care for adolescent contraception; a pelvic examination is not needed for provision of contraceptive services. When sexually experienced teens come in for *any* clinic visit, they should be given immediate services for contraceptive needs and screening for sexually transmitted infections (STIs). Since adolescent compliance is difficult to predict, *every opportunity should be used* to screen and educate the teen on sexual health and responsibility during every health visit and physical examination done for illness or well-care.

Confidential sexual health care must be available and should be provided. Laws in many jurisdictions permit teens to receive sexual health care without parental knowledge. This allows teens to get needed help in a non-intimidating way without the worry of embarrassment or censure. It is proven to support quality of life, improve health outcomes, and decrease health care costs. Giving consent for treatment, as well as medical record and information release permission can only be provided by the consenting adolescent for special medical concerns as required by law, such as services pertaining to: family planning services (i.e. pregnancy, birth control), sexually transmitted infection (STI), HIV/AIDS, and alcohol/substance abuse and treatment. If an adolescent is below the age of general medical consent, special medical consent by the adolescent is required and the parents may not sign to release or review such medical information. The adolescent's expressed written consent is required to release them to any party (including parents). It may be necessary to have a process for teen confidential billing for those who request confidential services. All clinic staff, including those responsible for processing requests for release of medical records, should be aware of these issues.

There are confidentiality exceptions to information release if, for instance, the clinician believes that the circumstance is an emergency or dangerous situation, he/she may disclose the information to the parents after consulting with the adolescent or making a good faith effort to do so. Clinicians who have reviewed the adolescent's medical record may deviate from such policy when extenuating circumstances warrant disclosure of selected information, and when it is in the best interest of the adolescent (i.e. the teen is dangerously non-compliant or missing).

Components of a Sexual History
- Number of sexual partners (currently and total lifetime number)
- Partner age and length of relationship

- Gender(s) of sexual partner(s)
- Gender identity and sexual orientation
- Types of sexual activity (vaginal, oral, anal intercourse)
- Last intercourse, with or without condom
- Frequency of intercourse (> two times per month needs more than foam and condom)
- Age at first sexual intercourse
- Whether patient or partner desires pregnancy
- Previous/current contraception
- Type of contraception desired
- Current understanding of contraceptive options
- Condom use: consistency and appropriateness of use
- Past history of sex without condoms
- Whether parent(s) are aware vs confidentiality (confidential billing and test results; cell phone or partner's telephone number)
- Current symptoms of STI
- Previous chlamydia test/last STI testing
- History of prior STI
- History of sexual abuse or exploitation
- History of exchanging sex for drugs or money
- Recent medications: OTC, Rx (oral acne antibiotics), herbal

Additionally for Females

- First day of last menstrual period (LMP)
- Regularity of menses
- Last pelvic exam, if any
- Past history of: hepatitis, diabetes, thrombosis in legs
- History of previous pregnancy. If pregnant, would keep or ITOP?
- History of sex without condom, or condom-accident since LMP
- Ability to remember to take daily pill

Current Cervical Cancer Screening Recommendations

The 2009 update of evidence-based cervical cancer screening recommendations for cervical cancer screening (Pap testing) is based on the low incidence of cervical cancer under age 21, the long duration necessary for progression of disease, that 70% of sexually active teens will get human papillomavirus (HPV), that low grade SIL will not progress to high grade for 5 years, that 97% regress in 3 years, and that low grade SIL does not require culposcopy for 2 years. As of November 20 2009, the American

College of Obstetricians and Gynecologists (ACOG) recommends that first cervical cancer screening be delayed until age 21. It was stated that all women should have their *first cervical cancer screening at age 21* and can be re-screened less frequently than previously recommended, according to newly revised evidence-based guidelines issued November 20 2009 by ACOG and published in the December 2009 issue of *Obstetrics and Gynecology*. Less frequent tests are now recommended after age 21; most women from age 21–30 should undergo cervical screening once every 2 years instead of annually.

A Pap test (and a pelvic exam) for healthy adolescents under age 21 is now an unnecessary invasive procedure which deters teenagers from getting STI screening and obtaining contraceptive services. Urine STI screening and contraception counseling should begin immediately after first intercourse.

Parenthood Desire and Sexual Experience

Personal psychological needs create ambivalence and a desire for a baby in nearly 1 out of 5 American teens: an achievement, having love, relationship security, independence and freedom, replacing a loss. A clinician should not expect that a sexually active adolescent who has ambivalence or a desire for a baby will be compliant with contraception. Three-quarters of those who desire parenthood had sexual intercourse, compared to 38% of those who do not ($p < 0.001$). Females who feel very overweight had measurably more desire to parent ($p = 0.002$); males did not ($p = 0.35$) [Paperny, 1997].

Some Psychological Concepts of Ambivalence and Desire for Pregnancy
- If it happens, it happens.
- I want to get pregnant.
- I want to be sure I *can* get pregnant.
- I want someone to love and someone who will love me.
- All my friends have babies.
- All women have babies; it's natural.
- Why not make a baby? My mother says she wants to be a grandmother.
- Having a baby would make me want to finish school.
- I want a place of my own.
- I don't mind if I get pregnant.
- If I get pregnant, my boyfriend won't break up with me.
- My boyfriend won't let me use birth control.
- My boyfriend makes me have sex.
- My boyfriend wants me to get pregnant.

Sexual Experience

About half of all secondary-school-aged adolescents in the United States have been sexually active (are sexually experienced), and about one-third are ongoing sexually active. In the United States, the median age of first sexual intercourse is 16.5 years old. These data vary by country, race and cultural norms. Whether adolescents report being sexually active on interview, being *sexually experienced* is strongly associated to significant risk for negative consequences of sexual activity including pregnancy and sexually transmitted diseases. About a third of adolescents report being pressured to have sex. The younger the onset of sexual activity, the more likely there was coercion. Sexual activity often occurs with other risk behaviors such as substance use. Approximately one-third of young teens report doing more than they intended sexually because of alcohol or drug use, and 1 in 5 did not use condoms because of use of these substances.

When discussing sexual activity with an adolescent, consider a variety of behaviors other than vaginal intercourse, such as co-masturbation, oral sex, and anal sex. A third of females and nearly half of males in secondary school have had oral sex and half consider it to be less important than sexual intercourse. Many engage in oral sex to avoid intercourse and consider oral sex to be a form of "safer sex". Sexual experience increases with age; a third of 15-year-olds and two-thirds of 18-year-olds report sexual experience.

Sexually Experienced Adolescents

by Age	13	14	15	16	17	18	19
% Males	13	22	34	52	60	62	79
% Females	11	25	39	51	63	72	79

(42 % of all teens had sexual intercourse) [Paperny, 1997]

Only about 1 in 5 American youths have had sexual intercourse prior to age 15, with 3% of females and 7% of males being sexually experienced by age 12. Reasons given by younger teens for having sex: wanting to feel grown-up, curiosity, partner pressure, and friends having sex. For older teens, the reasons are: being in love, having a partner who was drunk or high, physical attraction, and feeling romantic. Partner age difference affects the sexual behavior of younger female teens; 11% of females had a partner 3 or more years older. Sexual experience increases as the age difference between the partners increases. For same-age partners, 13% of relationships include intercourse, but when the partner is at least 3 years older, 33% involve intercourse. When there is a large age difference between partners, it is more likely sex is involuntary. Also, a younger age at first intercourse makes it more likely that sex is unwanted or involuntary. One in 8 females who had sex at age 14 or less say it was involuntary.

Adolescent Pregnancy

In most developed countries, the rates of adolescent sexual activity are similar, and most Western countries have open communication and discussion about sexuality issues which facilitates access to contraceptives for sexually active teens. The exception is the United States, which still has the highest rate of teen pregnancy, and where teens are less likely to use contraceptives and use them effectively. This is partly due to sexual mores of the country as well as political attitudes. For instance, abstinence-only programs (which have been promoted in the United States in recent years) significantly increase the number of pregnancies among partners of young male participants: Relative risk = 1.54 (95%, CI: 1.03–2.29). Such programs have a paradoxical effect on teen pregnancy [DiCenso *et al.*, 2002].

There are long-term socioeconomic disadvantages for pregnant teens, including lack of advancement in education, poverty, and poor outcomes in emotional and social development of their children. Pregnant teens under age 16 are more likely to have delayed prenatal care, inadequate weight gain, and higher rates of pregnancy-associated complications, including depression. After teen pregnancy, a third of adolescent mothers will have a second child in 1 year and a quarter will have a second child within 2 years.

Conditions Associated to Pregnancy in Adolescents Under the Age of 15 Years
- Preterm birth.
- Higher post-neonatal mortality rates.
- Low birth weight (four times more than other ages).
- Sudden infant death syndrome (SIDS) (three times more than other ages).
- Congenital malformations (1.5 times more than other ages).

Laboratory Diagnosis

When testing a teen for pregnancy, always ask in advance about her plans if her pregnancy test is positive. Since some teens want to become pregnant, this should be known in advance. The beta subunit of human chorionic gonadotropin (hCG) will identify a pregnancy about 10 days after fertilization, just around the next missed menstrual period. False negative urine tests are rare. Repeating a negative test in 2 weeks is sometimes warranted (but begin contraception immediately if feasible). Home pregnancy tests should be confirmed with a clinical test.

After diagnosis of pregnancy, the adolescent should be informed confidentially of the positive result. Feelings about the pregnancy are discussed. If the adolescent is a minor, discuss her plans for telling her parent(s) and the conceptive father. If the adolescent desires to terminate the pregnancy, then the clinician should confidentially assist the patient when feasible, and provide future contraception. However, it is the clinician's discretion to inform pregnant minors who desire a baby and who are living at home, that parental involvement will eventually be necessary. It is important to get a sense of the expected parental response from the patient. Timing is particularly important if the teen is a dependant whose parents will eventually learn about the pregnancy and hold the clinician responsible for not involving them in a timely manner in pregnancy termination or management, as well as parental responsibility for payment for the medical expenses of prenatal care and delivery (and grandparenting!). If the parent is present, or if the parent can come to an office visit in a few days, the teen may find it easiest to tell a parent with the physician present if a very negative response is anticipated.

Fetal sizing and gestational dates should be determined (often by ultrasound), and unbiased counseling should include the options of parenthood, adoption (not commonly completed), and pregnancy termination. Most jurisdictions have specific laws regarding abortion for minors. In the United States, 9 out of 10 abortions are performed during the first trimester of pregnancy, with half done in the first 8 weeks. Adolescents should otherwise begin prenatal care as soon as possible to help prevent negative outcomes; counseling is necessary on proper diet and non-use of alcohol and drugs.

Contraception

Consistent use of contraception is required to prevent pregnancy. Some teens are poorly motivated to avoid pregnancy as previously discussed. Other obstacles to regular use are that contraception is equated to a high interest in sex, and that spontaneity is "limited" by contraceptive planning. Most contraception must be individualized. A supportive clinician can often motivate a teen to prevent pregnancy. In the United States, actual adolescent contraceptive use is often limited by misconceptions and psychological factors. Certain female adolescents who have been sexually active feel they are unable to get pregnant. There were 12% of girls who worried that there was something wrong with them so they cannot get pregnant. Of these girls, 33% desired parenthood, compared to 9% of others ($p < 0.001$). Four out of 10 were having sex more often than every 2 weeks, and 55% were at high risk for pregnancy, compared to 11% of others ($p < 0.001$) [Paperny, 1997]. There are some teens, both females and their male partners, who believe that birth control is not safe: in one study, 34% of males and 29% of females felt that birth control pills and shots are unsafe [Paperny,

1997]. For these and other reasons, including availability and cost, actual adolescent contraceptive use is limited.

Adolescent Contraceptive Use (Males and Females)
Frequency of use: 31% always, 23% sometimes, 46% never.

Method used	%M	%F
None	6	34
Withdrawal or rhythm method	12	18
Condom and/or foam	28	18
Birth control pills/shot	(19)*	25
Other	5	5

(*partner) [Paperny, 1997]

   Clinicians should review psychological factors and desires as well as choices for contraceptive options available and help the patient decide which method he or she would be most likely able to use properly and consistently. Clinicians should also emphasize the need to protect from STIs and human immunodeficiency virus (HIV) as well as pregnancy, and to use dual methods that include latex condoms. It is necessary to address confidentiality and parental involvement, as well as payment for the medical visits and the contraceptive. Parental involvement is useful since adolescents are more likely to be successful with their method if their parents are aware and supportive of use of contraception. If confidentiality cannot be guaranteed or there are financial issues, the adolescent should be referred to a free public clinic. Health education and counseling should include that the mortality rate from pregnancy and childbirth for all women under age 30 is far greater than for women using any form of contraception, including abortion. Oral contraceptives (OC) or medroxyprogesterone acetate/Depo-Provera (Depo) have been estimated to be as much as nine times safer than pregnancy for adolescent girls. There are significant health benefits of hormonal contraceptives. Depo can decrease the frequency of grand mal seizures and sickle cell crises.

Health Benefits of Hormonal Contraceptives (particularly oral)
• Relief from dysmenorrhea/less cramps and spotting.
• Decreased menstrual flow/less iron deficiency anemia.
• Reduced premenstrual syndrome (PMS) symptoms.
• Reduced rates of endometrial cancer (50% less).
• Reduced rates of ovarian cancer (40% less).
• Decrease in ovarian cysts (50–80 % less).
• Reduced rates of fibroids (30% less).
• Reduced development of fibrocystic breast changes/benign breast lumps.
• Decreased gonococcal pelvic inflammatory disease (PID).

- Suppression of endometriosis.
- Improved HDL/LDL cholesterol levels.
- Improved menstrual migraines.
- Improved acne (some OCs).
- Improved bone density.

There are six contraceptive methods that are most feasible for the majority of teens and young adults. All teens need to know about these: 1. Abstinence (sometimes feasible), 2. Non-coital sex (oral and anal carries STI risk), 3. Condom with foam (reasonable for coitus less often than every 2 weeks), 4. Oral contraceptive pill (requires compliance, parent discoverable), 5. Depo (invisible, requires compliance to return to clinic), and 6. Emergency contraception (Plan B within 5 days of unprotected intercourse).

Contraceptive Use Effectiveness for Teens (if consistently used)

- Abstinence 99%.
- Depo 98%.
- OC 91%.
- Condom and foam 90%.
- Condom 85%.
- Foam 75%.
- Withdrawal 50%.
  (Percentage of fertile couples using a method for 1 year that did not get pregnant)

Oral contraceptive pills (OC) and condoms are common methods used worldwide. All low dose OCs are safe and effective in healthy adolescents. A pelvic examination is not necessary prior to prescribing hormonal contraception, and there is no need for a physical examination in most patients, only the need to obtain a sexual history, blood pressure and a chlamydia urine test. There are few, rarely present, contraindications to use of hormonal contraception in healthy female adolescents. Chronic illness is not necessarily a contraindication. Clinicians should emphasize use of two methods (condom + hormonal contraception) to protect from STIs and HIV infection as well as pregnancy.

The Male Condom

The male condom is probably the most universally used contraceptive worldwide. The advantages of the condom as a contraceptive are that there are virtually no side effects, no prescription is needed and the latex condom provides some protection against STIs, while being 85% effective contraception. It also allows the male to share responsibility for contraception and may prolong coitus by delaying ejaculation. There is reduced incidence of cervical cancer, and the condom can assist in relieving dyspareunia. It is important to counsel that condom use with contraceptive foam, sponge or insert increases efficacy, and that oil-based lubricants are contraindicated with latex condoms because of increased failure and breakage. Oil-based lubricants can be used with those made out of polyurethane.

Reasons Given by Adolescents for Not Using a Condom as a Contraceptive
• Decreased penile sensation.
• Need to disrupt foreplay to put it on.
• Stigma of use associated with promiscuity.
• Stigma of use associated with STI.
• Failure of physicians to advocate it.
• Failure of pharmacists to display openly.
• Need for proper use technique to prevent failure.
• Cost and availability.
• Religious beliefs.
• Unwillingness of some males to accept responsibility for contraception.

Medroxyprogesterone Acetate Injection (Depo-Provera)

The medical history, the blood pressure and weight are the only elements necessary before hormonal contraception is prescribed; a gynecologic examination and/or Pap test are not needed. Fear of the pelvic exam has long been a deterrent for adolescents to obtain contraceptive services. Patients with a family history of thromboembolism should be evaluated for thrombotic disorders before starting hormonal contraception containing estrogen. Detection of STIs can now be done easily by urine DNA-probe testing, and is preferred. If the history suggests possible pregnancy, a urine pregnancy test is performed before prescribing hormonal contraception. Clinicians may administer the first Depo shot within 5 days of the beginning of menses or simply do a pregnancy test before giving the injection. Depo patients with prolonged amenorrhea should be evaluated for pregnancy by the clinician after 2 weeks, or at 11 weeks when seen for the next injection. None of the hormonal methods are teratogenic, and if pregnancy is discovered after starting a method, there is no concern about harm to the fetus.

There are many advantages to the use of Depo for adolescents. It does not interfere with sex, and is private and invisible. There is no need to take a daily pill, and is as effective as being sterilized (if given on time). About a third of adolescents appreciate the convenience that the menses stop (after they get past the worry of amenorrhea from pregnancy). Depo use is safe and effective to provide at the time of testing and counseling [Hatcher, 2003], and family history of DVT is not a contraindication for Depo (WHO Medical Eligibility Criteria for Starting Contraceptive Methods). Depression also is not a contraindication for Depo [Westoff *et al.*, 1998], and the use of Depo does not affect breast cancer risk [Westoff, 2003]. The concern about bone density loss is mediated by the fact that it is reversible [Kaunitz, 2005] and adolescents who stop using Depo can increase their bone density to comparable levels as their peers (calcium supplements and vitamin D is preventively recommended).

The cost for Depo is approximately the same as that of OCs. Depo is given as 150 mg intramuscularly (IM) every 11 weeks. (Scheduling 1 week earlier than the recommended 12 weeks allows for a week of tracking and follow-up of those adolescents who do not show up for their appointments). There is no teratogenic risk to a developing fetus if already pregnant. Early recommendations were to give it within 5 days of menses, but it is best to give it immediately regardless of menstrual cycle day if an hCG is negative at the visit. In that case, a repeat hCG before the next dose is recommended. The contraceptive effect is within 24 hours (unless given close to ovulation), and fertility usually returns in 12 weeks to 12 months following last injection. It is important to preempt concerns about side effects, since about a third of patients will have menstrual spotting or irregular unpredictable bleeding (inconvenient), and a third will have amenorrhea, both of which will generate worries about danger of use. Only a third have the same menstrual cycle. Giving earlier doses of Depo (if spotting is toward the end of 11 weeks) or adding estrogen-containing OCs for a few months can alleviate menstrual spotting, which often resolves by itself after a few Depo doses. Two other intolerable side effects (which also require preemption) are weight gain (more than that from OC) and mood changes. Counseling about healthy caloric nutrition and exercise is critical.

Oral Contraceptives

For adolescents starting oral contraceptives (OCs), it is best to prescribe a 28-day monophasic pill so there is no stopping when dosing the pill. The most convenient is to start OCs on Sunday after the next menses (so that menses begin on the last Tuesday). If adequate testing and follow-up for possible pregnancy is feasible, then immediate start of OC can be done regardless of menses. The contraceptive effect occurs within 7 days, so contraceptive foam with condom use is recommended for 7 days. Ovulation may occur if pills are taken late, so a *12-hour grace period* is usually acceptable. If a pill is 12 hours late, take the late one immediately, then foam and condom use is recommended for 5 days.

OC Contraindications

- History of thrombotic disease.
- Active acute or chronic liver disease.
- Poorly controlled diabetes mellitus or seizures.
- Undiagnosed Hypertension >160/100.
- Severe migraines with focal neurological symptoms.
- Certain structural heart disease.
- Breast cancer and estrogen-dependant neoplasia.
- Known pregnancy (though no fetal injury occurs).

OC failure rate may be as high as 15% in teens because of inconsistent use, and some studies show they miss about three pills per month. There is no significant weight gain with low dose OCs. Some females may experience fluid retention. Breakthrough bleeding may occur in the first few months and then usually resolves. It is common if the patient is missing pills, and may also suggest an STI. Most patients have regular menses after a few months. Smoking is not a contraindication to OC, although WHO recommendations are to use 20 mcg of ethinyl estradiol for heavy smokers. Mini-pills are progestin-only and have decreased efficacy compared to estrogen-containing OCs. Those taking the Mini-pill should do so at the same time every day.

Possible OC Side Effects (very individual)

- Depression, mood changes, fatigue.
- Nausea or increased appetite and mild weight gain.
- Tender breasts.
- Elevated blood pressure.
- Acne (sometimes improved).
- Vascular HA (sometimes improved).
- Thrombosis (rare).

Emergency Contraception

All adolescents should be informed about the availability of emergency contraception (EC). Less than 10% of American women know about Plan B. In the United States, Plan B could eliminate up to half of the 3 million unintended pregnancies and nearly 1 million abortions. To prevent pregnancy, EC is the use of hormonal medication after unprotected sex, but can also include emergency insertion of an IUD. EC containing only progesterone reduces the risk of pregnancy by about 90%, and those with both estrogen and progesterone reduce the risk by about 75%. Once a pregnancy is established, EC is ineffective and will not disrupt an existing implanted pregnancy. EC does not increase risk of ectopic pregnancy,

EC Advantages
- Can be used even if patient cannot take regular birth control pills.
- There is no teratogenic risk to a developing fetus if already pregnant.
- Even thromboembolism is *not* a contraindication to Plan B.
- Efficacy of Plan B: 85%, if taken within 5 days after unprotected intercourse.

The common progestin-only method is called Plan B (Levonorgestrel 0.75 mg and the newer double-dose pill). It is best given within 72 hours of unprotected intercourse, but to some extent, it is effective for up to 120 hours. The original two-dose Plan B (Levonorgestrel 0.75 mg) was previously given as two doses 12 hours apart, but now both pills should be given simultaneously. Plan B One-Step 1.5 mg as a single double-dose pill is now available. This progestin-only method is well-tolerated and produces little nausea and vomiting. Only 23% have nausea and 6% vomiting, but there is no need to give an anti-emetic since vomiting implies that adequate medication was already absorbed. There is no need to re-administer a vomited dose unless the patient gagged and vomited while swallowing pills. There are no contraindications to giving EC (except allergy to it) and they are available without prescription in many jurisdictions.

Clinicians should give adolescents a standby prescription so that they can have it readily available to use soon after unprotected intercourse. Provision of a prophylactic supply increases use five-fold, which is why recommendations made by major professional organizations include routinely offering a prescription to all reproductive-age females and to all postpartum women. Combination OCs can also be used as EC. They should contain ethinyl estradiol and levonorgestrel; multiple pills should be given as two doses 12 hours apart in multiples so each dose is equal to 100–120 micrograms of ethinyl estradiol and 0.50–0.75 mg of levonorgestrel. When an estrogen-containing EC is given, an anti-emetic may be needed.

Obtain an hCG if no menses occur within 4 weeks after an EC dose. Every patient should see a provider within a month for contraceptive counseling and planning. Ideal adolescent contraception (besides abstinence) is *triple protection,* that is condom + hormonal contraception + Plan B. Anticipatory discussion about potential side effects of the chosen contraceptive method is crucial to success, as well as a process available for adolescents to contact the clinician to ask questions. Adequate communications to troubleshoot problems will prevent adolescents from quitting their contraceptive. Regular clinician follow-up every few months maintains compliance and provides the opportunity to manage concerns.

Other Contraceptives

Other contraceptives which may be used in adolescents include the subcutaneous implant, intrauterine device (IUD), patch, and vaginal ring. The best results are those that do not require daily or coital-dependent compliance. IUDs have a low failure rate, but have often been avoided in adolescents because of concerns about risk of STIs and pelvic inflammatory disease (PID); the risk is only a concern in those with multiple sexual partners. The risk of PID is at the time of insertion, and it does not increase simply because an IUD is in place. Implanon (the subcutaneous implant) is used in circumstances requiring extraordinary efficacy for extended periods of time. The transdermal contraceptive patch has better compliance than OC with comparable efficacy but there is 60% more total exposure to estrogen and should not be used in adolescents weighing over 90 kg due to risk of pregnancy. Vaginal hormonal ring contraception (NuvaRing) is complicated for young adolescents since it is inserted into the vagina and left there for 3 weeks, then removed during the fourth week for menses; if it is expelled or out for over 3 hours, back-up contraception is required for 7 days. Vaginal barrier contraceptives (diaphragm, cervical cap, and the female condom) have rather limited usefulness for adolescents due to high failure rate and difficulty of use. There is also an increase in urinary tract infections (UTIs) in diaphragm users.

Health Care for Gay, Lesbian, Bisexual, Transgender, and Questioning (GLBTQ) Youths

During adolescence and young adulthood, issues of sexual orientation are dealt with on a conscious level and self-identification of sexual orientation becomes clearer. A significant number of youths are now dealing with these issues, and significant morbidity and mortality is associated with being lesbian, gay, or bisexual (LGB) in every society. The failure of physicians to discuss sexual orientation with their patients has resulted in thousands of lost and injured lives. Research shows many American college students who self-identify as gay, lesbian, or bisexual knew about their sexual orientation in high school and some were even aware in grade school. Adult surveys show that 3–10% of the American population is gay or lesbian. Studies of adolescents suggest that 1–5% consider themselves as bisexual, gay, or lesbian but 1–10% are "unsure" about themselves. With increasing age, more adolescents and young adults self-identify as homosexual. Adolescence is a stage of development that reflects experimentation, change, and growth. Often, no absolute conclusions can be made about an adolescent's sexual orientation at this time of life. Many experts believe that a person's sexual behavior is not a totally accurate indicator of his or her true sexual orientation and that more important clues in that regard are provided by a detailed history of the individual's sexual feelings and fantasies. Many GLBTQ youths are only heterosexually active or not sexually active at all. The homosexual-heterosexual continuum must be separately evaluated in terms of the person's behaviors (action or practice) and feelings (preference or arousal).

Eventually, it is possible to distinguish between a lifelong pattern of homosexual contact versus a developmental interlude of adolescence. Studies of homosexual and heterosexual adults reveal that homosexual contacts are common in the early life of both groups [Schofield, 1965]. Most individuals who manifest some homosexual behavior during pre-adolescence and adolescence will not develop into adult homosexuals. Homosexual contact peaks between the ages of 11 and 15, and only 6% of girls report homosexual experiences, compared to 11% of the boys [Sorenson, 1973]. For the majority, this interlude seems to be a testing of emerging sexual feelings, and may be a response to curiosity, anxiety, or concerns about normalcy. For others, it is a manifestation of their deepest sexual orientation.

Variations in Sexual Development

Few health professionals have a complete understanding of the variety of developmental possibilities that comprise the complexity of human sexuality. One's sexuality includes gender identity, gender role, and sexual orientation [Green, 1974].

Three Components of Sexual Identity
- *Core morphologic gender identity* (essence) reflects a self-recognition as male or female and begins early in life, usually before age 2. It is the internal acknowledgement of being either male or female.
- *Gender-role behavior* (practice) begins in the ensuing years, as most children begin to act like other children of his/her sex. It is the overt outward expression of being male or female.
- *Sexual-partner orientation* (preference) occurs in late adolescence or young adulthood, when the individual chooses partners with whom to engage in socio-sexual relationships.

Heterosexual individuals are attracted to (and prefer over time) the opposite sex, homosexual to the same sex, and bisexual to both sexes. In most cases, gender identity and role coincide with the individual's anatomic sex. Transexuality (transgender) describes individuals who feel that their core gender is different than their biologic sex, which is different from transvestism (cross-dressing transvestite) where one simply dresses in clothes of the opposite gender. Transgender individuals and transvestites can be heterosexual, homosexual, or bisexual. Transvestites may dress in the clothes of the opposite gender for erotic or non-erotic psychological reasons. It is usually a male who has male core morphologic gender identity and is heterosexual in regard to sexual preferences. Surveys of adult transvestites reveal that approximately half began cross-dressing prior to puberty and about half began cross-dressing during adolescence. The sexual-object choice of a transsexual individual is the same biologic sex, but since the transsexual does not actually feel that he is a member of this sex in a true sense, he or she should not be considered a homosexual.

Sexual orientation is established by very early childhood and it is not volitional for the individual. Gender identity may be determined before birth. Biological and/or environmental determinants are not fully understood, but twins tend to similar sexual identity, and there has been clustering within family pedigrees [Stronski-Huwiler, Remafedi, 1998]. There is also a possible relationship with prenatal hormones. There is no evidence that parenting issues, abuse, or other causes relate to homosexuality. Furthermore, sexual orientation does not always coincide with an individual's actual sexual practices — individuals who self-identify as heterosexual may engage in sexual activity with those of the same sex, and those that self-identify as homosexual may be sexually active with individuals of the opposite sex.

Stages of Homosexual Identity Acceptance
- Stage 1: Sensitization (perceptions of being different from peers)
- Stage 2: Identity Confusion (during puberty: homosexual feelings lead to inner turmoil)
- Stage 3: Identity Assumption (during or after late adolescence)
- Stage 4: Commitment (same sex relationships more open, disclosure and "coming out" increases)

The progressive acceptance of a homosexual identity in adolescence occurs over time; this is not a "decision" made as a single life event. Approximately 4 years separate the mean age of the beginning of ongoing homosexual experiences and the point of self-designation as homosexual.

	Average Age	
	Females	Males
First awareness of homosexual attractions	14–16	13
First homosexual experience	20	15
Self-identification as lesbian/gay	21–23	19–21

Issues for GLBTQ Youths

A major problem for GLBTQ teenagers is the lack of adequate and appropriate role models. While older adolescents may have available a wider group of acquaintances for socializing, the younger adolescent frequently finds himself alone or is relegated to a social life of youth discos and juice bars where the street-youth subculture may promote promiscuity, drugs, and prostitution. A professional who is engaged in counseling this group of adolescents should be aware of and recommend constructive community resources supportive of GLBTQ youths.

The process of "coming out" usually denotes a progressive revelation of homosexual orientation to others who are close [DeMonteflores, Schultz, 1978]. Parental approval is important to all adolescents, and since most societies (including many family members, friends, and acquaintances) will not be accepting of this disclosure, the adolescent may feel very isolated, lonely and be subject to depression. Often, it is at this time that school or job performance declines. For the adolescent who is in school in certain countries, there may be much harassment to the point that the adolescent quits school. A number of youths are referred by parents for help at this time.

Risks to Gay, Lesbian, Bisexual, and Transgender Youths
- Suicide.
- Substance use and abuse.
- STIs, including HIV.
- Dropping out of school.
- Being thrown out of their homes and living on the street.
- Sexual activity including coercive sex.
- Disordered eating.
- Body image dissatisfaction.

The sequelae of GLBTQ youths' experiences of isolation, fear and violence include: family conflict, school failure and drop-out, risk-taking (sex, drugs, prostitution), conflict with the law, depression, and suicide. Homosexual adolescents may be 2–3 times more likely than their peers to attempt suicide, and account for as many as 30% of completed teen suicides each year [Paperny, 1997; Stronski-Huwiler, Remafedi, 1998].

Clinical Issues

"Any physician who believes she/he has no LGB teens in her/his practice is not asking the right questions." — Robert Bidwell MD

Issues to Address with a GLBTQ Adolescent

- Developing a good practitioner-patient relationship.
- Evaluation of sexual orientation and gender identity (sexual history).
- Evaluation of relations with peers, family and at school.
- Medical considerations related to sexual behaviors.
- Experiences of violence at home, at school, in the community.
- Thoughts of self-harm.

Clinical Approach to GLBTQ Youths

Clinicians may be confronted with a teenager who announces his or her homosexuality, but it is most common that an adolescent will not announce to the clinician that they are GLBTQ. One must assume patients could be "straight" or "gay," and use gender non-specific questions, and listen for gender non-specific answers. Stereotyped assumptions must be avoided. All sexually active females are not heterosexual. A young woman who is not having sexual intercourse is not necessarily celibate. A masculine-appearing male adolescent may not be heterosexual, nor an effeminate-appearing male adolescent homosexual.

Developing rapport with adolescents who may be homosexual can be more difficult than with heterosexual adolescents. The practitioner's attitude may favor one kind of lifestyle over another but should not be brought into the clinical interview or influence patient management. Comments that may seem biased or non-accepting should be avoided. Ask if the adolescent is attracted to or has had sexual experiences with "men, women, or both". Use neutral nouns such as "lover" or "sexual partner" instead of "boyfriend" or "girlfriend".

A helpful written questionnaire might include an open-style question such as: *Do you have a boyfriend or girlfriend lover? Yes/No (If "Yes", circle which one).* The sexual history may be somewhat limited at the first discussion by GLBTQ adolescents who may not immediately want to be totally open. Discuss relationships and ask about signs/symptoms of STIs as well as pregnancy. Ask about use of "protection" and comfort with sexual activities. The clinician who can communicate genuine interest, understanding, and acceptance, regardless of sexuality, is likely to find that an adolescent who claims to be homosexual has probably not entirely accepted that and would welcome an opportunity to discuss the subject with someone whom he/she respects.

If, however, it is clear that the adolescent has very much accepted homosexual orientation, there are further considerations. Therapy to change orientation is ineffective. Aversion therapies to change sexual orientation are psychologically destructive and unethical. The important task is to determine the degree of conflict that sexuality poses for the adolescent. For many adolescents, the real need is to help with the adjustment to a same-sex orientation and the resulting challenges.

Many adult transsexuals desire to have sex-change/sexual reassignment surgery, at which time sex-object choice will be in line with anatomy. This is usually contraindicated in adolescence, for both medical-legal reasons and due to the emotional and developmental instability of these individuals in the adolescent age group. In both adults and adolescents, treatment of transsexuals with psychotherapy for changing core gender identity has been futile (and is unethical). There is often a great deal of personal pain and anguish that a young teenage male with ambivalent gender identity undergoes during this developmental period associated with maximal sexual frustration. There is frequently a crisis when secondary sexual characteristics arise (deepening of voice and increased facial hair) that are dissonant with his identity in the feminine role as he is rendered less and less capable of passing as a woman. Some older adolescents who spend most of their time dressed as the opposite sex and request surgical sexual reassignment should be considered for hormonal therapy. The male transsexual, when dressed as a woman, is most at ease and behaves more naturally, and his behavior is feminine rather than effeminate.

Medical Management

The medical needs of GLBTQ adolescents are all the same as other teens — with some additions. And, there are no sexual activities or behaviors that are specific to LGB teens. All GLBTQ youths need validation, acceptance, and medically accurate information. It is always helpful to explore and address prejudice, discrimination, harassment and "coming out" issues. The clinician should address resources to reduce isolation, look for signs of abuse and neglect, and do specific tests according to anatomic site exposure risk, gender, and sexual habits (e.g. oral GC culture, anal GC culture, or even anal Pap test). Discussion should include safer sex, gay-bashing, suicide prevention, and issues of sexual assault survivors (4 times incidence in LGB youth). There is no need to report a teen's sexual orientation to parents, and it can possibly do great harm. Clinicians should be careful with documentation and know the clinic's policy on release of medical records to families.

For male to female transgender youth, hormonal therapy has tremendous psychological value and may decrease the very strong desire for surgical sex change. Some breast growth and the knowledge that female hormones are circulating in the bloodstream may allow him to feel he is on the way to becoming a woman. One regimen that has been suggested for males is 0.2–0.4 mg of oral ethinyl estradiol per day [Hembree *et al.*, 2009]. Alternatively, estradiol valerate or cypionate 5–40 mg every 2 weeks can be given IM. An anti-androgen such as spironolactone may be given at 200–400 mg/day. Breast and prostate examinations should be done regularly, and liver function tests are often appropriate. For female to male transgender youth, hormonal therapy is often testosterone enanthate or cypionate usually given at 100–200 mg IM every 2 weeks [Hembree *et al.*, 2009; Futterweit, 1998].

The clinician can best help adolescents with cross-gender orientation by general exploration of all sexual options, attending to all issues of adolescence, being supportive to the adolescent, and providing reassurance to the parents. When needed, work with the families of LGB youths to facilitate understanding and acceptance. Referral to experienced supportive community resources can include individual counselors, teen and parent support groups, books, brochures, teen lines, Internet sites, and specialty clinics. Advocacy is useful through residency programs, professional societies and academies, schools, churches, and legislatures.

Female Reproductive Disorders

Amenorrhea

Primary amenorrhea is the lack of menarche by age 16, or by stage Tanner 5, or if it has been over 4 years from the start of Tanner 2 without menarche. Secondary amenorrhea is defined as 6 months or missing three cycles in a row in females that previously had menses. Irregular menses are normal up to 2 years after menarche due to anovulatory cycles (with no corpus luteum producing progesterone, unopposed estrogen secretion causing negative feedback in the hypothalamic-pituitary axis, and subsequent decreased estrogen levels causing endometrial shedding).

The Differential Diagnosis of Amenorrhea
- Pregnancy
- Anatomic: imperforate hymen, transverse vaginal septum, agenesis of cervix, uterus, vagina, uterine synechiae, pituitary tumor
- Hypothalamic: tumors, gonadotropin-releasing hormone (GnRH) deficiency, familial, chronic or systemic illness or stress, athletics, eating disorders
- Endocrine: pituitary, ovarian (including genetic/chromosomal), polycystic ovary syndrome (PCOS), adrenal, thyroid, contraception

Pregnancy can present as primary or secondary amenorrhea depending on age of onset of sexual activity. Clinicians must always consider pregnancy as a cause of secondary amenorrhea, and must not forget pregnancy as a possible cause of primary amenorrhea. Polycystic ovary syndrome (PCOS) has oligomenorrhea or amenorrhea with signs of elevated androgens including virilization, acne, hirsutism, and clitoromegaly and can be associated with dysfunctional uterine bleeding. Athletic amenorrhea comes from strenuous exercise causing hypothalamic-pituitary axis dysfunction and amenorrhea; up to two-thirds of all athletes may have this condition. Clinicians should recognize the female athlete triad: amenorrhea, osteoporosis, disordered eating. Since osteoporosis increases the risk of stress fractures, there is more risk for athletes in sports preferring a light body build, such as ballet dancers, runners, and gymnasts.

Evaluation includes a history to identify chronic illness, and an examination looks for signs of endocrine problems suggesting thyroid or adrenal disease, pubertal development including the stage and sequencing and the timing of puberty, and whether menses are expected at the pubertal stage. Genitalia are examined for clitoral enlargement and a patent hymen. The vaginal opening is easily assessed by inserting a small, moist cotton-tip swab into the vaginal opening. A vaginal-abdominal or recto-abdominal examination determines the presence of the uterus and cervix. A pelvic ultrasound will best define upper tract anatomy. MRI of the head with views of the sella can rule out prolactinoma. A pregnancy test and thyroid-stimulating hormone (TSH) test should be done.

In the case of finding no etiology for secondary amenorrhea, then do a progesterone challenge with 10 mg oral medroxyprogesterone daily for 10 days. If withdrawal bleeding occurs, then the problem is with anovulation (stress, drugs, exercise, PCOS). If no bleeding occurs, do estrogen/progesterone cycle test or refer for further evaluation. If there is withdrawal bleeding and high LH/FSH with estrogen/progesterone cycle, the problem is ovarian failure. If withdrawal bleeding occurs with low or normal LH/FSH, then there is possible CNS lesion or hypothalamic dysfunction. If no withdrawal bleeding occurs, refer for further evaluation for Asherman syndrome.

Dysfunctional Uterine Bleeding (DUB)

Treatment should palliate the acute bleeding, and evaluation should determine if there is a treatable underlying cause of the bleeding (e.g. STI, pregnancy, PCOS/endocrine, hematologic, systemic illness, foreign body like a tampon). If the bleeding is otherwise mild, and the patient has normal hemoglobin, the cycle can be observed by following a menstrual calendar. Iron supplements can often prevent anemia and antiprostaglandin medication may help. In moderate DUB, a combined OC (estrogen and progestin) is most effective and preferred. Hospitalize patients with severe DUB and hemoglobin less than 8 gm/dL, or those with orthostatic changes.

Dysmenorrhea

Dysmenorrhea is pain associated with menses, which 20–90% of adolescents may experience. Primary dysmenorrhea is menstrual pain not associated with pelvic pathology, but rather with ovulatory cycles which cause smooth muscle contractions and associated symptoms such as vomiting, diarrhea, and dizziness. Other symptoms can include headache and backache. Secondary dysmenorrhea is menstrual pain from pelvic pathology such as endometriosis, uterine/genital tract malformations or obstruction, and PID. Medical history should include family history of endometriosis and the severity of pain, including any inability to go to school or participate in daily activities. Patients with mild symptoms and improvement with non-steroidal anti-inflammatory drugs (NSAIDs) can simply have an examination of the external genitalia to ensure patency of the hymen, but a pelvic examination will better define the anatomy. Laboratory tests for STIs and pregnancy should be done for sexually experienced adolescents. The use of NSAIDs, taken immediately with the onset of menses, can block the effects of prostaglandins. Ibuprofen and Naproxen are commonly used, but if inadequate, adding OCs may help. Try Depo for those who cannot tolerate OCs or estrogen.

Premenstrual syndrome (PMS) is a group of symptoms that occur cyclically during the menstrual cycle and end with the onset of menstruation; 5–10% of females have symptoms that affect their daily activities. Diagnosis requires that symptoms occur for several cycles, not be caused by other physical or psychological problems, and both recur and disrupt activities. Premenstrual dysphoric disorder (PMDD) has more severe feelings of depressed mood, mood swings, anxiety, and anger or irritability that interfere with daily activities. Treatment for PMS includes education, stress management, exercise, NSAIDs, spironolactone, and sometimes OCs or Depo. PMDD can be improved by selective serotonin uptake inhibitors.

PMS Symptoms
- Emotional: Irritability, fatigue, lethargy, insomnia, hypersomnia, depression, anger, mood swings, poor concentration, social withdrawal
- Physical: Headaches, leg or breast swelling, overeating, food cravings, weight gain, abdominal bloating, joint and muscle pain

Breast Disorders

Female adolescents may experience a number of problematic conditions, most of which include asymmetry, small or large size issues, pain, masses, and various nipple discharges. Breast masses in adolescents are almost never primary malignancies, but are almost always caused by a number of benign conditions. Painful masses are sometimes infections (often unilateral) or can be fibrocystic changes which occur during the menstrual cycle or with OCs. Ultrasound is sometimes useful to determine if a mass is cystic, but mammograms are not useful for adolescents. Breast self-examination has frequently been promoted for teenagers, but current recommendations are that breast self-examination should begin at age 35. Clinical time with adolescents should focus on more productive preventive services.

Male adolescents most often experience physiologic gynecomastia at early puberty (Tanner 2–4) which is benign, yet a common worry for teens and their parents. It usually resolves in about 2 years, but some teen males become very upset by having visible breast tissue, and request surgery (nearly always inappropriate). Physical examination of nipples, axillae and testicles is important; if the mass is not directly under the nipple, axillary nodes are present, or the patient is not Tanner 2–4, further workup may be indicated.

Male Reproductive Disorders

Urinary tract infection (UTI) is rare in a healthy male adolescent, and dysuria is commonly urethritis from an STI in a sexually experienced male adolescent. Any patient with only one testicle and the possibility of cryptorchidism is at risk for malignancy and should be referred to a urologist. Certain scrotal and testicular problems may be true clinical emergencies requiring immediate intervention, particularly testicular torsion. Teaching a testicular self-examination for cancer is a useful preventive measure since testicular cancer is the most common solid tumor in adolescent males, although rare.

Usually Painless Testicular Masses/Conditions
• Inguinal hernia.
• Varicocele (right-sided ones require evaluation).
• Hydrocele and spermatocele.
• Cancer.

Usually Painful Testicular Masses/Conditions
• Incarcerated hernia.
• Epididymitis/orchitis (requires STI evaluation).
• Torsion of testicle or its appendage.

Abdominal Pain

The complex list of conditions in the differential diagnosis of abdominal pain in adolescents is similar to that of younger and older age groups, but in this age group it is more often related to sexually transmitted diseases (STDs), PID and UTI. A basic abdominal pain workup should include a comprehensive history and physical examination, and a variety of laboratory studies including, but not limited to, a complete blood count (CBC), erythrocyte sedimentation rate, urinalysis, sometimes stools for occult blood as well as ova and parasite tests, and a pregnancy test for females.

Sexually experienced female adolescents should be tested for STDs and may require a bimanual pelvic examination to evaluate the possibility of subacute or chronic PID or other gynecologic conditions. Ovarian cysts, acute PID and adnexal torsion are the most common gynecologic causes of acute pelvic pain in adolescent females, while endometriosis is a common cause of chronic pelvic pain.

Urinary Tract Infection

UTI in females occurs more often during puberty, partly because of sexual activity as well as hygiene (females should have been taught to wipe downward after urination). Males have very few UTIs. The symptoms of UTI can be the same as those of vaginitis or STIs. There are three categories of symptoms of UTI: 1. Cystitis, with infection located in the lower urinary tract, 2. Pyelonephritis, where the infection includes the kidney (upper tract disease), and 3. The urethral syndrome, which is inflammation of only the urethra. The same bacteria found in the stool are found in the urine of UTI patients because of contamination of the urethra, then ascend up the urethra into the bladder, and sometimes into the kidney through the ureter. Vesicoureteral reflux facilitates retrograde flow and progression of infection upward.

Symptoms and Signs of Lower Urinary Tract Infection
• Dysuria
• Frequency
• Urgency
• Suprapubic pain
• Hematuria

Symptoms and Signs of Upper Urinary Tract Infection
• (Current lower tract symptoms may be absent; check recent resolved symptoms)
• Fever
• Flank pain
• Costovertebral angle tenderness

In sexually experienced adolescent males, symptoms of dysuria may actually represent urethritis from an STI rather than a UTI, and dysuria may be accompanied by urethral discharge. In females, STI pathogens (e.g. *Chlamydia trachomatis*, *Neisseria gonorrhoeae*, *Trichomonas vaginalis* and *Candida vaginitis*) can cause symptoms of lower tract infection, or may be the result of non-infectious causes of urethral irritation such as trauma from sexual intercourse. Remember that concurrent UTI and vaginitis or STI is common among sexually experienced females. To confirm lower tract UTI, rule out vaginitis, urethritis and non-infectious causes of urethral discomfort. (Many adolescents with STI have no signs or symptoms of genital infection.)

Evaluation and Treatment

STIs and UTIs often have the same presentation: frequency, urgency, abdominal pain, fever, and possible discharge. The treatment for a UTI may not cure the STI, but *symptoms may disappear.* That is why it is critical to do urine cultures for all adolescents when ordering a urinalysis and planning to only treat what appears to be a UTI (even though a "reliable" sexual history is obtained). Should the patient end up culture-negative, the clinician should at least order a follow-up urine Chlamydia trachomatis (CT) test. If no urine Neisseria gonorrhoeae (GC) test is available, it is feasible to obtain a vaginal GC culture by self-swab.

Pyuria is 95% sensitive and 70% specific and can represent both inflammation and infection; most adolescents with symptomatic UTI have pyuria. White blood cells (WBCs) in urine do not always indicate bacterial infection, and more importantly: *the absence of pyuria does not rule out infection.* Hematuria often occurs in acute cystitis, but this is not specific since hematuria occurs in other conditions.

Leukocyte esterase measures the enzyme contained in WBCs; it has a sensitivity of about 80–90% with a high specificity. False negatives occur. *Always do a urine culture on all adolescent patients; a negative culture suggests possible STI if those tests were not ordered.* Any male suspected of having UTI must have a urine culture prior to any treatment. It is obtained as a clean catch specimen and should be plated within 2 hours. A positive urine culture is defined as greater than 100,000 organisms per mL, but S. *saprophyticus* is a common UTI pathogen which presents with lower counts. Polymicrobial infection (three or more) usually represents contamination. Asymptomatic bacteriuria found on urinalysis is not significant and should not normally be treated, except in pregnancy. Upper tract infections can show leukocytosis on a complete blood count and an elevated C-reactive protein or erythrocyte sedimentation rate.

It is critical to test for STIs and vaginitis, even with a "seemingly reliable" history of no sexual activity. External genitalia examination can reveal trauma or other causes such as herpes simplex and other causes of vulvar ulcers. Testing should be done to look for CT, GC, *T. vaginalis*, bacterial vaginosis, and yeast. Radiologic studies are usually unnecessary, but they are indicated when there is recurrent pyelonephritis, lack of response to therapy, male gender, or suspicion of an underlying abnormality, such as obstructive uropathy, urolithiasis, or a complication of infection such as a renal or perinephric abscess. Renal ultrasound is frequently a first test to order because it is fast and is non-invasive. Voiding cystourethrogram can demonstrate vesicoureteral reflux and obstructions like posterior urethral valves.

The preferred treatment of lower tract infection is normally a 3- to 5-day regimen in uncomplicated cystitis in females, but 7 days of treatment are recommended for women with symptoms lasting for more than 1 week, pregnant women, men, and patients with complicated UTI in diabetes.

Sexually Transmitted Infections

Most STIs are asymptomatic in adolescents. All sexually experienced adolescent and young adult women should be screened at least annually for CT, regardless of whether they are considered "high risk". Recommendations for screening of males vary. Adolescents and young adults have the highest age-specific rates of infection.

Relative STI Prevalence in the Unites States
- Chlamydia 278
- Gonorrhea 128
- AIDS 15
- Syphilis 12

Asymptomatic females are much more likely than male adolescents to be tested for STIs during routine health visits or when they obtain reproductive health care and contraception. The presence of one STI should prompt the clinician to investigate for others; co-infection is quite common. By high school graduation, 1 out of 4 American teens acquire a STI.

Sexual activity at a young age creates high STI risk — they are limited at skills for negotiating sexual activity and condom use with partners, and substance use may cause young adolescents to engage in risky sexual behaviors. Also, younger adolescents are less capable of anticipating consequences of their decisions. Inconsistent or ineffective condom use and perceived barriers to confidential health care further increase the risk of having an STI, as does the high prevalence of ectropion in early adolescence.

STI Testing Recommendations
- All sexually experienced adolescent females should be screened annually for CT infection, and routinely screen for GC and *Trichomonas vaginalis*.
- For high risk adolescents (those with new partners, multiple partners, or history of a prior STI), screen for CT every 6 months, since reacquisition is common.
- Starting at age 21, Pap smears should be performed every 2 years to screen for cervical dysplasia caused by human papillomavirus (HPV).

- STI screening in adolescent males should include CT in those with a history of multiple partners and/or inconsistent condom use.
- A rapid plasma reagin (RPR) or Venereal Disease Research Laboratory (VDRL) test may be indicated, based on the local prevalence of syphilis infection and personal risk factors.
- Screening for human immunodeficiency virus (HIV) in adolescents whose behaviors place them at increased risk of this infection should be considered.
- Patients diagnosed with one STI should be screened for the presence of all others (including syphilis and HIV infection). When CT is found, testing for GC is mandatory. (When GC is found, treatment for CT is recommended.)
- Men who have sex with men should have routine tests for: HIV and syphilis, urine/urethral testing for GC, urine/urethral testing for CT, pharyngeal culture for GC in men with oral-genital exposure, and rectal culture for GC and CT in those who have had receptive anal intercourse.

Only *culture* for GC is the appropriate test for rectal and pharyngeal specimens, not other testing forms. Otherwise, nucleic acid amplification tests are available for both GC and CT; they include polymerase chain reaction (PCR), ligase chain reaction (LCR), and sensitivities range from 85–99%, with specificity 97–99%. DNA from the pathogenic organism may persist in the vagina for several weeks following successful treatment; it is therefore recommended that retesting only be done after 6 weeks have elapsed. Convenient urine specimens allow for STI screening without performance of a speculum examination or urethral swab.

Treatment approaches must include education; patients should be educated about their infection and its natural course, any need for follow-up testing, and their personal risk factors for future STIs, and how to decrease the risk. Single-dose medications are available for the treatment of several STIs. Advantages of single-dosing include high patient compliance, the ability of the provider to document witnessed treatment, and the need for a test of cure is eliminated due to high efficacy. Patients should abstain from sexual contact until both patient and partner have completed therapy. Condom use should be recommended for every sexual encounter, but explain that it does not always prevent catching an STI. Discuss sexually risky behaviors, elimination of certain sexual partners, and the possibility of abstinence as a means of avoiding STI. Sexual partners within the past few months should be told, either by the patient, the clinician, or the health department, that they may have been exposed to an STI. Partners should be instructed to obtain testing and treatment for the STI. Some clinicians prescribe treatment for both the patient and the partner.

STI Diagnosis and Treatment

Chlamydia (CT) is the most common bacterial STI and the most common reportable infectious disease in the United States; surveillance reports more than 1 in 10 female adolescents at school-based clinics are positive for CT. Females between 15–19 years old have the highest incidence of infection, followed by those between age 20–24. Again, *all* sexually experienced females under 25 years old should be screened annually for CT. Order a urine CT test for a female if she is sexually experienced and was not tested in the last 6–12 months, had any intercourse without condoms in the last 6 months, has a new sexual partner, or is sexually experienced and presents with signs or symptoms of UTI. CT infections are usually asymptomatic in both males and females, so appropriate screening of males is also indicated. Females may present with cervical or vaginal discharge, urethritis, or PID. Almost half of untreated infections progress to symptomatic PID. Males may have non-GC urethritis (half of which is caused by CT) or epididymitis. Culture for CT has a low sensitivity (75%), but antigen detection techniques and DNA probes have better sensitivity and are more easily processed. Treatment for uncomplicated cervicitis or urethritis may be Azithromycin 1 g orally (single dose) or Doxycycline 100 mg twice daily for 7 days. (Alternative: EES 800 mg orally qid for 7–10 days or Erythromycin base 500 mg orally qid for 7–10 days). Those with PID or epididymitis require additional therapy. Test of cure is not always necessary, but repeat chlamydia testing should be no sooner than 6 weeks after treatment. Most patients should be retested in a few months, since re-infection is common. It is not necessary to treat all patients with CT infections for GC, but they should be tested for it (obtain a long intravaginal swab for gonorrhea testing).

Neisseria gonorrhoeae (GC) infection of the lower genital tract may cause purulent vaginal, cervical, urethral, or rectal discharge, dysuria, and local discomfort. Ascending infection can cause PID or epididymitis. However, GC may be completely asymptomatic, especially in females. After oral sex, the adolescent may contract GC pharyngitis, which is also usually asymptomatic. GC is a common cause of septic arthritis in adolescents, which mostly affects medium and small joints, and complaints of polyarthritis. Culture (with modified Thayer-Martin medium) is effective for the diagnosis of GC infections, with good sensitivity (85%). Amplified DNA probes have improved sensitivity, and the advantage is the use in testing urine specimens. Treatment may be a single-dose treatment for uncomplicated cervicitis or urethritis and includes: Cefixime 400 mg orally once, or Ceftriaxone 125 mg once intramuscularly, or Ciprofloxacin 500 mg orally (unless local quinolone resistance exists), or Ofloxacin 400 mg orally once. Also treat for chlamydia when treating GC, unless CT has been ruled out or tested, since over half of GC infections are also infected with chlamydia.

Herpes simplex virus (HSV) is the common cause of genital ulcers. HSV serotype 2 (HSV-2) causes 65% of those and has frequent recurrences. Up to 1 in 5 of sexually active young adults is sero-positive for HSV-2, and most are asymptomatic. Symptoms may be genital vesicles and ulcerations, inguinal adenopathy and sometimes systemic symptoms. Adolescents with HSV-2 may have six or more outbreaks a year during the first 2 years. Triggers for recurrence can include stress, menses, fatigue, or other illness. Prodrome may include tingling, itching, pain or burning at the sites of lesions. Although treatment with Acyclovir 400 mg orally three times daily for 7–10 days may help the acute episode, such treatment does not eradicate the latent virus, nor does it affect the frequency or severity of recurrences later. Twice-daily continual suppressive antiviral therapy may help those with more than six recurrences per year, and it can reduce transmission to others.

Human papillomavirus (HPV) is the *most common* STI acquired by adolescents. Probably half of females under 25 years old are infected, and about 75% of sexually experienced adults have serologic evidence of past infection. Certain serotypes are associated with squamous intraepithelial lesions (SIL) and invasive ano-genital cancers, and other serotypes are mostly seen as genital warts. In most infected people, the infection will resolve within 5 years (many within 1 year). High-risk serotypes are more likely to persist. Untreated genital warts may remain unchanged, spread, or resolve spontaneously, although this may take months or even years to happen. Asymptomatic HPV infection may surface as an abnormal Pap smear. Low-grade intraepithelial lesions frequently seem to follow new HPV infections, but most resolve spontaneously in adolescents. (Please refer to page 175: most recent Pap recommendations for females starting at age 21.) Genital warts are usually visually diagnosed and rarely require biopsy. Treatment involves application of caustic topical medications to lesions in the genital and perianal areas.

Early diagnosis and treatment of *human immunodeficiency virus* (HIV) infection may slow the decline of immune system function and decrease HIV-related mortality and morbidity. Persons with high-risk sexual practices should be strongly encouraged to undergo HIV testing. Patients should be informed that HIV testing may not detect infection acquired in the recent few months, as it may take a few months to become detectable by various test methods. Pretest and posttest counseling should be performed, and informed consent should always be obtained; some adolescents may prefer anonymous testing in public clinics. At the same time *syphilis* testing can be done, and positive syphilis patients may best be served by an infectious disease or STI specialist. Clinicians should know the features of acute retroviral syndrome, which may occur in the first few weeks following HIV acquisition. This mononucleosis-like syndrome is characterized by fever, adenopathy, malaise, and a skin rash; it occurs in about half of newly infected adolescents. During this time, *antibody tests such as*

EIA are not yet positive, so test HIV RNA by PCR for earlier identification; a positive test should be confirmed by a later test. Adolescents who are newly positive for HIV must receive initial counseling at the time of diagnosis. They should be reevaluated for the presence of signs or symptoms that suggest advanced disease. They also require psychosocial evaluation, risk-reduction counseling, and antiviral therapy. New patients may best be served by an HIV specialist, but all should be promptly referred for comprehensive medical, psychosocial, and mental health services.

Trichomonas vaginalis, caused by a flagellated protozoan, is an infection that often co-exists with gonorrhea or bacterial vaginitis, and is often asymptomatic, or shows a frothy vaginal discharge and mild vulvovaginal itching; mild dysuria may occur. Vaginal discharge is commonly grey-greenish with a "musty" odor; wet-mount microscopic examination of the discharge shows moving flagella of the parasite. Treat with metronidazole 500 mg orally twice a day for 7 days (or treatment with 2 g once may be adequate). Sexual partners should be treated, even if asymptomatic.

Bacterial vaginosis occurs mostly in sexually experienced adolescents and exhibits changes in the vaginal flora. Symptoms include a white vaginal discharge (often coating the vaginal wall), with a "fishy" odor, but is otherwise asymptomatic of abdominal pain or pruritis. Etiology is an increase in *Gardnerella vaginalis* and decrease in *Lactobacillus*. Microscopy shows Clue cells (squamous epithelial vaginal cells covered with bacteria). Treatment is Metronidazole 500 mg orally twice daily for 7 days or intravaginal gel 0.75% 5 g daily for 5 days. Be aware that a whitish cottage cheese discharge with microscopic hyphae and little odor but associated with pruritis and sometimes an erythematous rash may be *Candida* vulvovaginitis requiring clotrimazole or nystatin treatment.

Sex Education

Clinicians should communicate the following to adolescents: If you have ever been sexually active, get STI tested:

1. At least every year, *even* if you feel fine.
2. If you think you may have been exposed to a sexually transmitted disease.
3. If you didn't always use a condom.
4. If you have a new sex partner.

Clinicians may the only resource for adequate and accurate sexual health education and counseling: All teens need the awareness that he or she can be seen confidentially for sexual health services at the allowed age in the jurisdiction. It is usually optimal if a teen's parent can become supportive of the need for birth control and/or STI testing, especially to obviate need for confidential billing and payments. All adolescents need knowledge of the risks and benefits of the different birth control methods, risks of teen pregnancy and benefits of delaying pregnancy until young adulthood, benefits of sexual abstinence and the benefits of practicing safe sex. Multimedia and sex education computer games can facilitate attitudes and knowledge on these sensitive subjects [Paperny, Starn, 1989].

Sexual health education and counseling for females (and their partners) should inform that EC can be used as long as 5 days after a sexual encounter, that a pelvic examination is not a pre-condition for provision of contraception, and that the usual start time of contraceptive pills or shot is optimally at time of menses. They need to know when to return for pregnancy testing, i.e. if menses are 2–3 weeks late (unless taking Depo and not late for injections).

Common Sexuality Misconceptions
- The more an adolescent knows, the more likely he/she is to get into trouble.
- The best way to prevent immorality is to scare them.
- Abstinence-only programs help prevent teen pregnancy.
- Adolescents already know so much these days, why bother?
- Access to birth control will stimulate adolescent sexuality.
- By providing confidential access to contraception and STI tests, we are violating parents' rights.
- Sexually explicit educational material is pornographic.

Sexuality Facts All Adolescents Should Know
- Parenthood is neither desirable nor inevitable for everyone.
- Sexual thoughts and fantasies are normal.
- Masturbation is normal for children, adolescents and adults.
- Various kinds of foreplay are normal.
- Penis size varies, and worries are a waste of time.
- Pornography is (usually) not harmful; it is an alternative to sex, not a stimulant.
- STIs can be serious without treatment.
- Pregnancy can be avoided.

Sexuality Health Education Websites

www.SexEtc.org
www.GoAskAlice.columbia.edu
www.SIECUS.org
www.PlannedParenthood.org
www.Not-2-Late.com
www.ItsYourSexLife.com

A clinician who emphasizes responsible sexuality, provides sex education and general counseling can, thereby, be instrumental in helping the adolescent through a sometimes difficult period of development.

Suggested Readings and Bibliography

Adams Hillard PJ, Deitch HR. (2005). Menstrual disorders in the college age female. *Pediatr Clin North Am*, 52, pp. 179–197.

American Academy of Pediatrics. (2006). *Red Book: 2006 Report of the Committee on Infectious Diseases*. 27th Edn. (American Academy of Pediatrics, Elk Grove Village).

American Academy of Pediatrics, Committee on Adolescence, Blythe MJ, Diaz A. (2007). Contraception and adolescents. *Pediatrics*, 120, pp. 1135–1148.

Benjamin H. (1969). For the practicing physician: Suggestions and guidelines for the management of transsexuals. In: Green R, Money J (eds), *Transsexualism and Sex Reassignment*. (Johns Hopkins Press, Baltimore).

Bartle N. (1999). *Venus In Blue Jeans: Why Mothers and Daughters Need to Talk About Sex*. (Dell Publishing, USA).

Centers for Disease Control and Prevention, Workowski KA, Berman SM. (2006). Sexually transmitted diseases treatment guidelines, 2006. *MMWR Recomm Rep*, 55, pp. 1–94.

Deisher RW, Paperny DM. (1982). Variations in sexual behavior of adolescents. In: Kelley VC (ed), *Brenemann's Practice of Pediatrics*, Vol. 1, Chap. 25 (Harper & Row, Philadelphia).

DeMonteflores Z, Schultz SJ. (1978) Coming out, similarities and differences for lesbians and gay men. *J Soc Issues*, 34, pp. 59–72.

DiCenso A, Guyatt G, Willan A, Griffith L. (2002). Interventions to reduce unintended pregnancies among adolescents: systematic review of randomized controlled trials. *BMJ*, 15, 324 p. 1426.

Eisenberg L. (1969). A developmental approach to adolescence. In: Bernard HW (ed), *Readings in Adolescent Development*, pp. 55–62. (International Textbook Co., Scranton).

Emans SJ, Brown RT, Davis A, Felice M, Hein K. (1991). Society for Adolescent Medicine Position Paper on Reproductive Health Care for Adolescents. *J Adolesc Health*, 12, pp. 649–661.

Frankowski BL; American Academy of Pediatrics Committee on Adolescence. (2004). Sexual orientation and adolescents. *Pediatrics*, 113, pp. 1827–1832.

Fraser AM, Brockert JE, Ward RH. (1995). Association of young maternal age with adverse reproductive outcomes. *N Engl J Med*, 332, p. 1113.

Futterweit W. (1998). Endocrine therapy of transsexualism and potential complications of long-term treatment. *Arch Sex Behav*, 27, pp. 209–226.

Gold MA, Sucato GS, Conard LA, Hillard PJ; Society for Adolescent Medicine. (2004). Provision of emergency contraception to adolescents. *J Adolesc Health*, 35, pp. 66–70.

Green R. (1974). *Sexual Identity Conflict in Children and Adults*. (Basic Books, New York).

Greydanus DE, Rimsza ME, Matytsina L. (2005). Contraception for college students. *Pediatr Clin North Am*, 52, pp. 135–161.

Haffner D. (1999). *A Parent's Guide to Raising Sexually Healthy Children*. (New Market Press, USA).

Hatcher RA. (2003). *Managing Contraception 2003–2004*. 6th Edn. (Bridging the Gap Foundation, USA).

Hembree W, Cohen-Kettenis P, Delemarre-van de Waal H, *et al.* (2009). Endocrine treatment of transsexual persons: an Endocrine Society clinical practice guideline. *J Clin Endocrinol Metab*, 94, pp. 3132–3154.

Hillard PJ. (2005). Overview of contraception. *Adolesc Med Clin*, 16, pp. 485–493.

Kane ML, Rosen DS. (2004). Sexually transmitted infections in adolescents: practical issues in the office setting. *Adolesc Med Clin*, 15, pp. 409–421.

Kaunitz AM. (2005) Depo-Provera's black box: time to reconsider? *Contraception*, 72, pp. 165–167.

Klein JD, American Academy of Pediatrics Committee on Adolescence. (2005). Adolescent pregnancy: current trends and issues. *Pediatrics*, 116, pp. 281–286.

Mulcahey KM. (2005). Practical approaches to prescribing contraception in the office setting. *Adolesc Med Clin*, 16, pp. 665–674.

Paperny D. Aono JY, Hammar SL, Lehman R. (1989). Computerized evaluation of parenting desires, sexual and health behaviors, and pregnancy risk. *J Adolesc Health Care*, 10, p. 259.

Paperny D. (1997). Computerized health assessment and education for adolescent HIV and STD prevention in health care settings and schools. *Health Educ Behav*, 24, pp. 54–70.

Paperny DM, Starn JR. (1989). Adolescent pregnancy prevention by health education computer games: computer-assisted instruction of knowledge and attitudes, *Pediatrics*, 83, pp. 742–752.

Paperny D, Hicks R, Rudoy R. (1981). Chlamydial pelvic inflammatory disease in Adolescents. *J Adolesc Health Care*, 2, pp. 139–142.

Rickert V, Tiezzi L, Lipshutz J, León J, Vaughan RD, Westhoff C. (2007). Depo Now: preventing unintentional pregnancies among adolescents and young adults. *J Adolesc Health*, 40, pp. 22–28.

Rimsza ME. (2002). Dysfunctional uterine bleeding. *Pediatr Rev*, 23, pp. 227–232.

Rimsza ME. (2003). Counseling the adolescent about contraception. *Pediatr Rev*, 24, pp. 162–169.

Schofield MG. (1965). *Sociological Aspects of Homosexuality: A Comparative Study of Three Types of Homosexuals*. (Little, Brown & Co., Boston).

Shafii T, Burstein GR. (2004). An overview of sexually transmitted infections among adolescents. *Adolesc Med Clin*, 15, pp. 201–214.

Sorenson RC. (1973). *Adolescent Sexuality in Contemporary America*. (World Publishing, New York).

Spigarelli MG, Biro FM. (2004). Sexually transmitted disease testing: evaluation of diagnostic tests and methods. *Adolesc Med Clin*, 15, pp. 287–299.

Stronski Huwiler SM, Remafedi G. (1998). Adolescent homosexuality. *Adv Pediatr*, 45, pp. 107–144.

Timmreck LS, Reindollar RH. (2003). Contemporary issues in primary amenorrhea. *Obstet Gynecol Clin North Am*, 30, pp. 287–302.

Warren MP, Vu C. (2003). Central causes of hypogonadism — functional and organic. *Endocrinol Metab Clin North Am*, 32, pp. 593–612.

Westhoff C, Truman C, Kalmuss D, Cushman L, Davidson A, Rulin M, Heartwell S. (1998). Depressive symptoms and Depo-Provera. *Contraception*, 57, pp. 237–240.

Westhoff C. (2003). Depomedroxyprogesterone acetate injection (Depo-Provera): a highly effective contraceptive option with proven long-term safety. *Contraception*, 68, pp. 75–87.

Suggested Websites

Parents and Friends of Lesbians and Gays (PFLAG): http://www.pflag.org

Go Ask Alice! is a health Q&A site for older teens and college-age youth from the Columbia University Health Service. It provides in-depth, straight-forward, and non-judgmental information to assist young people in decision making about their physical, emotional, and spiritual health. Topics include relationships, sexuality and sexual health, emotional health, fitness and nutrition, tobacco, alcohol and other drugs, eating disorders, and general health: http://www.GoAskAlice.columbia.edu

Planned Parenthood Federation of America (PPFA) is committed to service, advocacy, education and research on human reproduction and sexuality. In addition to public policy and political action news, this site offers a variety of fact sheets and brief reports of interest to both professionals and the public. Topics include emergency contraception, chemical abortifacients, relevant Supreme Court rulings, and teen pregnancy statistics, among others. Consumer guides in both English and Spanish are also on line and cover topics such as reproductive health, birth control, abortion, STIs, help for teens, and guides for parents. PPFA's publications list, a roster of regional affiliates, and an extensive links page are available as well: http://www.plannedparenthood.org

TeenWire is sponsored by Planned Parenthood Federation of America. This site provides teens with uncensored and unbiased sexuality and sexual health information. This is drawn from both PPFA's own resources and from material submitted by teen peers (after review by PPFA). Teen site visitors are also encouraged to ask their own questions and to contribute their opinions and ideas. Some of the issues covered include changing bodies, choosing abstinence, protecting against sexually transmitted infections, preventing pregnancy, and establishing relationships: http://www.plannedparenthood.org/teen-talk

SIECUS develops, collects, and disseminates information on human sexuality, promotes comprehensive education in the field, and advocates the right of individuals to make responsible sexual choices. Annotated bibliographies, the current issue of Advocates Report, fact sheets on adolescent sexuality issues, parents' publications (some in Spanish), and other related information are all available online: http://www.siecus.org

FOCUS on Young Adults, for Youth In Developing Countries is a Pathfinder International program in partnership with The Futures Groups International and Tulane University School of Public Health and Tropical Medicine. Its goal is to improve the health and well-being of young adults in developing countries through the creation and strengthening of effective reproductive health initiatives. Information about the program, a series of four-page briefs on educational issues in young adult reproductive health, and a training module are online: http://www.pathfind.org/site/ PageServer?pagename=MAJOR_PROJECTS_FOCUS

SEX, ETC. is a teen-oriented newsletter from Rutgers University's Network for Family Life Education and produced by a teen editorial board with professional supervision. The newsletter is also published in a hardcopy edition three times a year and distributed free. (Bulk copies are available to adults who work with teens.) The current issue is online, as is a library of other topics, a Q&A section responding to all those questions teens want answers to but are reluctant to ask, and a recommended reading list. Some of the subjects covered include relationships, sexual decision making, abstinence, condoms and birth control (with limited detail as to precise use), drugs, alcohol and tobacco, gay and lesbian teens, pregnancy, and violence and abuse. The message is uncensored, non-judgmental, and unbiased: http://www.sexetc.org

MTV sponsored information: http://www.ItsYourSexLife.com

Emergency Contraception website is operated by the Office of Population Research at Princeton University and the Association of Reproductive Health Professionals, and has no connection with any pharmaceutical company or for-profit organization. This website is peer reviewed by a panel of independent experts: http://www.Not-2-Late.com

Chapter 8

Orthopedic Conditions and Sports

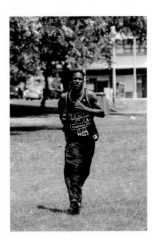

Overview

Only orthopedic conditions which are unique to the adolescent age group (including scoliosis, slipped capital femoral epiphysis and overuse syndromes in sports) will be discussed in this chapter. Syncope is included here since it may be related to participation in sports activities. Most non-sports-related injuries of adolescents are traumatic accidents, and many of those are head injuries resulting from vehicular accidents, including falls off bicycles. Many adolescents in secondary school participate in organized sports activities, and college athletics are popular worldwide.

Preparticipation Sports Evaluation

The Preparticipation Sports Evaluation (PSE) determines whether an adolescent is qualified to safely participate in a particular sport. The evaluation detects disqualifying conditions, and some primary care clinicians may not be experienced in detecting them. A clinician trained in sports evaluation doing so in the primary care setting is optimal, since the clinician usually already knows the adolescent. The history is the most important part of the PSE, and it detects past events that suggest conditions that could result in sudden death with exercise, including syncope with exercise or early cardiac death in an immediate relative. Past records of existing medical conditions should be reviewed. Review of previous injuries determines if they are not fully rehabilitated. It is important to check for a history of previous concussions and chronic conditions such as asthma.

Adolescent female athletes are particularly at risk for amenorrhea, osteoporosis, and disordered eating, especially those in gymnastics, long-distance running, and ballet. Take a history of oligomenorrhea and restrictive eating behavior. Amenorrhea in a female athlete should initially be evaluated with a sexual history and a pregnancy test when indicated.

History Questions for the Preparticipation Sports Evaluation
- Syncope or chest pain with exercise.
- Past concussion.
- Problems with any paired organs.
- Extremity injuries.
- Illness and chronic conditions.

The physical examination done at the PSE should include measures of height, weight, and blood pressure, and also Tanner stage is assessed by direct observation or by asking adolescent patients to point to pictures of stages of development that match theirs. The examination focuses on the cardiovascular system and on assessment of musculoskeletal integrity, strength, and flexibility, as well as the examination of paired organs. If hearing or vision is unilaterally impaired or if one kidney or testicle is defective, then disqualification for contact sports is usually necessary to protect the remaining functional organ. If a heart murmur is detected, evaluation needs to exclude a problem with a risk of sudden death, which may even require referral to a cardiologist. The most common cause of sudden cardiac death in young athletes is hypertrophic cardiomyopathy, which is usually inherited and causes a murmur best heard when the patient rises from a squatting position. Diagnostic criteria for Marfan syndrome include: tall stature with long limbs and fingers, pectus excavatum, and mitral valve prolapse, among others. Assess the strength of body parts essential to the particular sport, since that can decrease risk of injury. The PSE is a great opportunity to assess overall adolescent health when done by the primary care clinician. This opportunity is often the only one the clinician may have to accomplish comprehensive biosocial preventive screening and anticipatory guidance. A scoliosis screening should be done for all adolescents who have not finished their growth.

Scoliosis

Scoliosis, by definition, consists of a lateral curvature of the spine generally greater than 10 degrees. Idiopathic scoliosis, most common in adolescence, affects about 1 in 200 people with moderate to severe curves beyond 20 degrees. It usually develops in early adolescence, and the cause remains unknown though it occurs more frequently in some families. Mild curves of 20 degrees or less occur in 80% of cases and are distributed equally between males and females. Curves measuring more than 20 degrees occur much more commonly in females with a female to male ratio of 6 to 1. These curves require attention because they may progress and require treatment. Progression occurs primarily during the period of female peak height growth, just prior to menarche.

Primary screening for idiopathic scoliosis is done by visual inspection of the spine, looking for asymmetry of the shoulders, scapulae or hips. The clinician must discriminate whether a curve is structural or functional. Functional curves may be from poor posture or from other musculoskeletal causes such as leg length discrepancy. Additionally, with the adolescent bending forward at the waist, the clinician, observing from behind, looks for a unilateral rib hump. The scoliometer, a simple tool used in the office to measure tilt in the spine, provides another screening method. Patients with a visible curve, or greater than 5 degrees on the scoliometer, require a standing spine radiograph to quantify the curve and to serve as a baseline for any future progression.

Treatment of idiopathic adolescent scoliosis depends on patient age, magnitude of curve, and curve progression. Immature females with curves of 20 degrees or more are at highest risk for progression and should be referred to an orthopedist. Curves less than 20 degrees in a female who is Tanner stage 1–3, require follow-up exam and radiographs every 6 months to assess curve progression. A curve progression of five degrees or more should be referred to an orthopedist. In a more mature female at Tanner stage 4 or 5 that has reached menarche, curves up to 30 degrees have little risk of significant progression. More significant curves, however, should be referred, as well as patients with atypical curves or symptoms such as convex curves, pain, neurological findings, or bladder or bowel dysfunction.

Large curves, or curves with documented progression, may require bracing or surgical correction. In progressive curves measuring between 20–40 degrees, the use of a brace until bony maturity may prevent further progression. Patients with progression in spite of bracing, those non-compliant with bracing, and those who present with curves greater than 40 degrees may require surgical intervention.

Kyphosis

Kyphosis, or hunchback, consists of an accentuated forward curve of the spine beyond the normal 40 degrees. Severe or progressive kyphosis, like scoliosis, may require bracing or surgery. Generally, surgical correction of kyphosis should be considered in curves exceeding 75 degrees. Many teens exhibit a kyphotic appearance known as postural kyphosis which results from poor posture or slouching. Postural kyphosis will respond to education and exercise and does not lead to spine deformity. Structural or Scheuermann's kyphosis (with radiograph irregularity of the apophyseal growth areas of the thoracic vertebrae) results in kyphosis due to vertebral body wedging. Scheurmann's kyphosis may require treatment ranging from observation, exercise, bracing, and surgery, depending on the severity and progression of the deformity, as well as the presence of symptoms such as pain.

Syncope

Syncope is a transient, unexpected loss of consciousness and muscle tone from decreased cerebral perfusion, followed by spontaneous recovery without resuscitation. Healthy teenagers may faint in certain situations, and it most often occurs in middle adolescence. Any condition that decreases cerebral perfusion (including metabolic and psychiatric ones) can cause syncope. There are *vasovagal*, *cardiac*, and other *non-cardiac* causes of syncope. Vasovagal syncope is most common and usually precipitated by one or more of the following: *dehydration*, prolonged standing, arising quickly with postural hypotension, acute illness, anemia, as well as with such situations as pain, fear, anxiety, exhaustion, hunger, overcrowding, or seeing blood. Sympathetic response is followed by a parasympathetic one. Cardiac causes of syncope should be considered when it occurs *during exercise or while lying down*.

History should be obtained from both the adolescent patient and available witnesses. Ask about the last food and drink, medications, illicit drug use, time of day, the situation preceding the event, including position of the patient, and if triggered by exercise. Assess any associated symptoms such as the presence of chest pain, palpitations, seizure, pregnancy, injury, emotions, aura, fatigue, diaphoresis/sweating, headache, shortness of breath, visual changes, hearing changes, nausea, emesis, or ataxia. Inquire about duration of episode, loss of consciousness, appearance/status just after event, and a family history of sudden death, arrhythmia, congenital heart disease, seizures, or metabolic disorders. Most physical examinations for adolescents with syncope are entirely normal. Look particularly for cardiac and neurologic signs and symptoms. Blood pressure should he obtained with the patient supine and after standing for 10 minutes.

Differential diagnosis of Syncope

- Neurogenic/vasovagal: orthostatic, vasodepressor, reflex, autonomic
- Cardiac: aortic outflow obstruction (exercise, +/− murmur), PPHN, PE, MS, PS, myocarditis, pericarditis, atrial myxoma, tamponade, dysrythmia, prolonged QT
- Endocrine: hypoglcemia, electrolyte imbalance
- Toxic: CO, drugs
- Neurologic: syncopal or atypical migraine headache, seizure, hysterical, dizziness and vertigo
- Neuropsychiatric: hyperventilation, breath holding, narcolepsy, hysteria

Dizziness often precedes syncope, but can also be related to *vertigo*. A dizziness symptom diary is useful. Dizziness occurring with certain symptoms suggests potentially serious illness: with exercise, vomiting, a feeling that the room is spinning; headache or chest pain followed by syncope or loss of consciousness.

Common Orthopedic Conditions in the Adolescent

Today's adolescent population maintains a high level of participation in both organized and recreational sports and physical activity. As a result of this, many of their orthopedic conditions result from either acute injury (macrotrauma) or overuse injury (microtrauma) associated with these activities. Not all orthopedic conditions arising during adolescence, however, directly arise from physical activity. Slipped capital femoral epiphysis, although rare, is important because too often the diagnosis occurs late as a result of its sometimes confusing symptoms and a lack of awareness by the examining physician.

Slipped capital femoral epiphysis (SCFE) occurs as a result of posterior medial displacement of the femoral head at the proximal femoral growth plate. The slip may occur gradually or as an acute event. Often, an acute slippage occurs after a period of gradual slippage and chronic symptoms. A change in orientation of the growth plate of the femoral head and increased body size (or overweight) may cause gradual movement of the femoral head posteriorly and medially. Although relatively rare, occurring in less than 0.01% of pubertal adolescents, certain risk factors increase the prevalence — black, obese, prepubertal adolescent males have about a four-fold increased risk for

SCFE. It occurs bilaterally in up to one-third of patients. Patients with SCFE usually present with hip pain. The patient, however, may complain of only thigh or knee pain. Therefore, in any patient at risk for this condition, a complete examination of the hips, including radiographs, must be obtained in the setting of unexplained knee or thigh pain. There is usually a limp with a gait exhibiting the leg as externally rotated. Passive range of motion of the affected hip is limited, especially with internal rotation, flexion, and abduction. Assessing internal rotation with the hip flexed at 90 degrees is an effective screening maneuver, and should be done on all adolescents with lower extremity pain. Diagnosis is confirmed by anteroposterior and frog leg hip radiographs. Making an early diagnosis is very important for maintaining long-term function of the hip without arthritis. Providing early treatment prevents further slippage of the femoral head and avoids osteonecrosis and chondrolysis. Treatment in almost all cases involves surgical stabilization of the femoral head. SCFE must be ruled out in *any adolescent with an unexplained limp* so that detection and treatment are not delayed.

Patellofemoral pain occurs commonly in both the athletic and non-athletic adolescent. Most patients with patellofemoral pain syndrome experience anterior knee pain often associated with clicking, catching and locking. The pain occurs with activities that increase patellofemoral joint forces, such as kneeling, stair climbing and descending, deep squatting, and prolonged sitting. Commonly, knee pain is due to instability or anatomical abnormalities of the patellofemoral complex which includes the patella, the quadriceps muscle, the patellar tendon, and its attachment on the apophysis of the tibia. Often, there is dull, aching knee pain with no clear etiology. The patella seems the source of pain, but it may be in the surrounding area as well. As discussed earlier, in any adolescent with unexplained knee pain, the diagnosis of SCFE should be ruled out. Treatment includes activity modifications, ice, anti-inflammatory medication, and most importantly, a rehabilitation program directed at quadriceps strengthening, as well as a lower extremity stretching and strengthening program. Non-operative treatment has a high success rate. However, refractory patellofemoral pain may benefit from surgery directed at the underlying pathology.

Osteochondritis dissecans (OD) causes knee pain as a result of osteonecrosis of the underlying bone, then subchondral stress fracture. Although the exact cause of OD remains unknown, several factors including repetitive stress and a disruption of the blood supply to the bone appear to contribute to the condition. The most common site of this condition is the medial femoral condyle of the knee. The condition may progress from subchondral osteonecrosis with intact articular cartilage to articular damage and ultimately, formation of loose bodies, resulting in long term disability secondary to degenerative arthritis. Although symptoms usually present in late adolescence, the problem starts in childhood. Early diagnosis of OD during the time of growth is important because healing is possible at this stage. Pain and stiffness after running or athletic activities is the usual presentation. Later symptoms, such as joint locking, may indicate the presence of a loose body. The physical examination is usually not revealing, although there may be some swelling or quadriceps atrophy. Radiographs will usually reveal bony changes associated with OD. However MRI will provide a more accurate assessment of both bony and articular cartilage status.

Head Trauma

Most head trauma to adolescents is from injury resulting from vehicular accidents, or falls off bicycles without wearing a protective safety helmet. Since less than a third of adolescents using bicycles and skateboards wear helmets, promoting their use can prevent significant morbidity. *Concussion* is an alteration in cerebral function from brain trauma which may or may not involve loss of consciousness (LOC). About 1 in 5 secondary school football players have had a concussion, but less than 10% of concussions involve LOC. Clinical symptoms are usually functional disturbances, not structural brain injury detectable by scans. Headache and confusion are the most typical initial symptoms. Signs and symptoms of postconcussion syndrome are: amnesia, headache, dizziness, blurred vision, attention deficit, and nausea. If there has been concussion with LOC, an athlete should be removed from sports for at least a week and must be asymptomatic both at rest and with exertion in order to return. At a sports event where a concussion occurs, the athlete should have immediate cervical spine immobilization. If there is brief LOC (a few seconds), the athlete should be out of sports for a week, but if LOC lasts longer, or with repeated concussions, the athlete should stay out longer. Minimal brain injury is defined as head trauma with LOC lasting less than 30 minutes and post-traumatic amnesia lasting less than 24 hours. Because boxing produces repeated brain trauma, it is rarely recommended for young adolescents.

Urgent Referral is Needed when there is Head Trauma with

- Obvious skull fracture.
- Deterioration of mental status following trauma.
- LOC greater than 5 minutes.
- Focal neurologic signs.
- Persistent nausea/vomiting or headache.

Limb Injuries

Knee and ankle injuries account for greater than 25% of sports-related injuries in the adolescent. The majority of these injuries involves soft tissues and can be accurately diagnosed and treated by the general physician. Overuse injuries (from recurrent micro-trauma) occur more frequently in the younger athletic population. Older, more experienced athletes have fewer injuries than less experienced ones, partly because of attrition of injury prone athletes as well as improvements in conditioning and training techniques. Age may also determine the type of injury to an athlete. For example, a younger athlete with an open epiphyseal plate may experience a Salter-Harris fracture rather than a ligamentous injury as a result of joint trauma.

Traumatic injuries (i.e. sprains, strains, contusions and fractures) also occur frequently in the active adolescent. Initial treatment, particularly for soft tissue injury, utilizing the RICE approach (R-rest, I-ice, C-compression, E-elevation) should result in prompt resolution of symptoms. Cold packs should be applied intermittently for the first 48 hours for 30 minutes four times a day. Compression by an elastic bandage only assists in minimizing the amount of edema in the first 72 hours, and does not provide later protection or strength. The bandage should be worn for the first few days since edema can slow healing. Elevation reduces edema if the injured part can be raised to the level of the heart or above. Non-steroidal anti-inflammatory drugs (NSAIDs) or acetaminophen are the best anti-inflammatories and analgesics. Rehabilitation, after a brief period of rest, should aim at reducing inflammation, restoring joint mobility and muscular strength. Premature return to sports or physical activity commonly results in re-injury. Injuries accompanied by severe swelling, deformity, or inability to bear weight require further evaluation, including radiographs and orthopedic referral when appropriate. Similarly, injuries that do not respond to RICE promptly will also require further evaluation.

Acromioclavicular (AC) sprain, often called shoulder separation, occurs with a direct blow to the apex of the shoulder. The physical examination discloses tenderness over the AC joint and radiographs may reveal an increased distance between the acromiun and clavicle. Fracture of the *carpal navicular bone* can occur without initial radiographic findings. A high index of suspicion and appropriate follow-up X-rays will prevent late diagnosis of this injury and the occurrence of a non-union requiring surgery.

Ankle Sprains

Ankle sprains, the most common traumatic injury in the adolescent, comprise about a quarter of all athletic injuries. Although 80% of ankle injuries involve sprains, younger adolescents may injure the distal fibular growth plate. The most common mechanism of ankle injury, inversion, occurs in about 80% of ankle sprains and frequently involves damage to the anterior talofibular ligament. Physical examination should include an evaluation for localized tenderness and assessment of ankle stability. Suspected abnormal findings can be confirmed by examining and comparing the uninjured ankle.

Radiographs are not routinely required to evaluate ankle trauma. The Ottawa Ankle Rules provide a reasonable set of criteria to aid the provider in making a cost effective decision about the need for radiographs. Without using the Ottawa Ankle Rules, only about 15% of radiographs exhibit significant findings, and thus routine radiographs for all patients with ankle injuries is probably unnecessarily costly and time consuming.

Ottawa Ankle Rules for Evaluating the Young Adolescent with an Apparent Ankle Sprain

X-rays are only required if there is bony pain in the malleolar zone *and any one* of the following:

- Bone tenderness along the distal 6 cm of the posterior edge of the tibia or tip of the medial malleolus.
- Bone tenderness along the distal 6 cm of the posterior edge of the fibula or tip of the lateral malleolus.
- An inability to bear weight both immediately and in the clinic for four steps.

Ottawa Foot Rules for Evaluating the Young Adolescent with an Apparent Foot Injury

X-rays are only required if there is bony pain in the midfoot zone *and any one* of the following:

- Bone tenderness at the base of the fifth metatarsal.
- Bone tenderness at the navicular bone.
- An inability to bear weight both immediately and in the clinic for four steps.

Knee Injuries

Only 10% of knee injuries require surgery. Significant knee injuries commonly result in damage to ligamentous and meniscal (cartilage) tissue. The patellofemoral joint is also prone to injury in the adolescent. Anterior cruciate ligament (ACL) and medial collateral ligament (MCL) injuries represent the most common ligament injuries and may occur in isolation or as combined injuries. Approximately 50% of ACL injuries also involve a meniscal tear.

Female adolescents have three times the risk of ACL tears compared to males. The majority of these injuries occur as non-contact injuries in soccer and basketball.

Often, the athlete will experience a "pop" in the knee while pivoting on a planted foot or landing awkwardly. The athlete will often fall to the ground and be unable to return to play. A large effusion (hemearthrosis) usually occurs within hours of the injury. Once swelling has occurred, examination of the knee may prove difficult until the acute inflammatory process has resolved. The Lachman's test, performed at 20–30 degrees of flexion, provides the most reliable test of ACL integrity. The anterior drawer test, done with the knee in 90 degrees of flexion, is more useful to evaluate a chronic ACL tear. Radiographs of the knee following an ACL injury are usually normal. In most cases, the diagnosis of an ACL tear can be made on the basis of the history and physical examination. MRI will confirm the diagnosis but primarily serves to evaluate other intra-articular structures such as the menisci and articular surfaces. As with any acute injury, initial treatment with RICE will alleviate the initial inflammatory response. Referral to an orthopedic surgeon should take place at an early stage, both for confirmation of the diagnosis and because many of these patients will require ACL reconstruction if they plan to continue athletics.

The MCL is usually injured when there is an impact to the lateral side of the knee, creating a valgus force. Frequently, the athlete experiences a tearing sensation followed by medial pain, swelling, and stiffness. Physical examination will reveal tenderness over the MCL. Tenderness along the distal femoral physis, in the adolescent with open growth plates, suggests a physeal fracture. Severe medial instability of the knee, usually over 1 cm wide during a valgus stress test, suggests damage to the anterior and posterior cruciate ligaments as well. Since the MCL often tears along with the ACL, a high suspicion of ACL injury will decrease the chance of missing that diagnosis. Furthermore, although rare, knee dislocations can occur in the adolescent population and need to be considered when gross instability is present on examination. As with the evaluation of a suspected ACL injury, MRI will confirm the diagnosis and disclose additional intra-articular pathology. Injuries to the lateral collateral and posterior cruciate ligaments occur far less often than those to the ACL and MCL.

Meniscal injuries to the knee usually occur from rotation, hyperflexion, or hyper-extension injury. The medial meniscus, most commonly injured, has attachments to the MCL and should be considered with injuries to that ligament. Meniscal injuries often have tenderness on palpation of the involved joint line. In the McMurray test, pain or click upon external and internal tibial rotation while flexing the knee to 90 degrees, has about 60% specificity and sensitivity.

Overuse Disorders

Conditions such as patellofemoral pain syndrome, stress fractures, and Osgood-Schlatter's disease, result from chronic recurring stress causing microtrauma to anatomic structures. The intense, prolonged, repetitive training programs, which in the past were reserved for the elite athlete, are now often used by younger athletes with a resultant increased incidence of overuse injuries. As opposed to traumatic injuries, overuse injuries occur as a *process* not an *event*. The amount, intensity and frequency of exercise are major factors in the evolution of overuse injury. The affected body part is a result of the biomechanics of the sport (i.e. leg injuries are the rule in running-type activities), as well as personal variations of the athlete's anatomy (i.e. subluxating patella). The history of activity is key to making the diagnosis of overuse injuries. Often, the athlete has recently begun the sport or has markedly increased the training frequency, intensity or duration prior to the onset of symptoms. A change in training routine or improper training technique are also considerations: "too much, too soon, too fast." The relationship of the pain to the activity and the duration of the pain are indicators of the severity of the overuse injury and is the basis for the severity grading in the table below.

Severity of Overuse Injury

- Grade I: "soreness" after the sporting activity which resolves over several hours; there is no functional (performance) impairment and symptoms have been present less than 2 weeks.
- Grade II: pain that begins in the latter phase of the activity and persists after the activity; performance is not impaired and symptoms have often persisted for up to 3 weeks.
- Grade III: pain during and after the activity; performance is impaired and the symptoms have been present for up to 4 weeks.
- Grade IV: constant pain; symptoms are present over 4 weeks and performance is impaired so the athlete stops participating.

Osgood-Schlatter's disease, apophysitis of the anterior tibial tubercle, presents commonly in early and middle adolescent males with a tender, swollen anterior tibial tubercle (the site of insertion of the patellar tendon). As with most overuse disorders, treatment with RICE, activity modifications, and physical therapy will often effectively control symptoms. Rupture of the tendon from the tubercle is very rare, so athletic participation may continue based on toleration of pain. Patellofemoral pain syndrome (discussed earlier) is also a common overuse injury in adolescent athletes. *Stress fractures*, usually affecting the lower extremity, also occur as a result of overuse. Stress fractures of the proximal tibia are more than half of these types of injuries. Other stress fracture sites include the anterior mid-tibia (seen in jumping sports) and the metatarsals (of runners). Pain that persists for 3 weeks or longer and that occurs with weight bearing activities may indicate a stress fracture. Periostitis along the posterior medial tibia causes *shin splints*, which occurs with repetitive submaximal stresses seen in running and jumping. *Achilles tendonitis* occurs at the insertion of the Achilles tendon into the calcaneus.

Upper extremity overuse syndromes primarily occur in the elbow and shoulder. Adolescents involved in throwing sports such as baseball may develop overuse of the lateral elbow (lateral epicondylitis) or medial elbow (little leaguer's elbow). Adolescents involved in overhead activities such as throwing, swimming, and tennis, may develop overuse injuries of the shoulder. Primary disease of the rotator cuff, such as rotator cuff tendonitis and rotator cuff tears, does not commonly occur in the adolescent population. Secondary rotator cuff pathology, such as subacromial impingement, however, occurs commonly in throwing and overhead sports due to inherent gleno-humeral instability.

Other overuse injuries that affect the musculoskeletal system include spondylosis/spondylolisthesis, iliotibial band syndrome, and plantar fasciitis (which can be related to heel pain and Achilles tendonitis). Non-musculoskeletal examples of overuse injuries are sports anemia, exercise-induced amenorrhea and exercise-induced bronchospasm. Treatment of repetitive strain and overuse injuries requires specific patient education and can be prevented by appropriate training and supervision.

Many adolescents participate in weight lifting, either as a competitive sport such as powerlifting and bodybuilding, or as a means to improve their appearance or their performance in other sports. Weight training does not appear to have deleterious effects on the skeletally immature adolescent when performed using proper technique and safety precautions. Resistive strength training should begin with light resistance until proper technique is learned. Generally, resistance may then be increased to a level that allows the lifter to perform at least 10 repetitions. Adolescents should avoid competitive powerlifting, bodybuilding, and maximal lifts until they reach both physical and skeletal maturity. Nutritional counseling, particularly regarding the dangers of anabolic steroids, will help ensure the health and safety of adolescents involved in strength training.

Performance-Enhancing Substances and Techniques

Society values success, and adolescent athletes often look for the "edge" from supplements and drugs by using a variety of "potions", even when unsafe. *Anabolic-androgenic steroids* increase muscle strength and muscle mass, but are not proven to improve performance or endurance. They can cause aggressiveness, impaired judgment, impulsiveness, irreversible premature closure of growth plates, testicular atrophy, gynecomastia, acne, alopecia, hypertension, lipid abnormalities and multiple organ damage including malignancy. Compulsive use and withdrawal symptoms have been reported, and androgen use is punishable as a felony. *Androstenedione* (Andro, DHEA) may build muscle strength and poses the same risks as steroids when used in high doses. Stimulants like *ephedra* and *amphetamine* (addictive) delay fatigue and have multiple risks including sudden death. *Creatine* increases workout capacity and "water" weight of muscles, but does not increase muscle mass, strength or endurance. It is an expensive dietary supplement which may be helpful for enhancing muscle performance for high-intensity repetitive-burst sports; it can cause renal damage and other adverse effects if taken for more than a month. *Beta-Hydroxy-beta-methylbutyrate* (HMB) is a metabolite of leucine that may decrease protein catabolism creating a net anabolic effect. *Carnitine* is an amine found in meat that reduces muscle lactate accumulation and has no proven performance enhancement. *Chromium* is a trace mineral that decreases body fat and increases lean body mass.

Supplements may have contaminants and impurities and may not contain what the label states. Medical history should include, "Are you taking any medicines, vitamins or supplements?" Protein and amino acid supplements are expensive dietary supplements which could potentially increase muscle mass in the presence of a dietary deficiency and depend on the proper calorie and carbohydrate intake, but meat is more cost-effective to get the recommended 2 gm/kg/day! The *minerals* calcium and iron are important for female adolescents and are often underrepresented in the diet of the female adolescent athlete. Vitamin supplements are usually unnecessary in developed countries and a waste of money; excessive doses are harmful. A daily multivitamin with iron plus a form of extra calcium may be useful, particularly if the adolescent is not eating a well balanced diet. Calcium is necessary for bone strength and can be obtained from sufficient amounts of dairy products. Carbohydrate loading can create sluggishness and diarrhea. A pre-game meal of mostly complex carbohydrates should be eaten at least 2 hours before participation.

Fluid intake is most important for adolescent athletes. They must drink water at regular intervals during exercise, particularly with increased sweating in hot and humid environments where more fluids are needed. *Sports drinks* have simple carbohydrates and a good balance of sodium and potassium. Salt tablets are rarely needed and may be harmful as well as increase dehydration. Inadequate hydration during sports causes heat cramps, heat exhaustion, and heat stroke. The increased risk of such heat illness in hot, humid conditions is due to fast evaporation of sweat and the hindered loss of heat. Sports drinks also help to rehydrate after activity.

Other performance-enhancing techniques commonly used by professional athletes and Olympic competitors include: sufficient time to eliminate jet-lag after travel, getting 7 or more hours sleep nightly, relaxation and imagery training, self-hypnosis, and peak-performance training using both conventional and brainwave biofeedback.

Suggested Readings and Bibliography

Adirim TA, Cheng TL. (2003). Overview of injuries in the young athlete. *Sports Med*, 33, pp. 75–81.

American Academy of Pediatrics Committee on Sports Medicine. (1988). Recommendations for participation in competitive sports. *Pediatrics*, 81, pp. 737–739.

American College of Sports Medicine, American Dietetic Association and Dietitians of Canada. (2000). Nutrition and athletic performance. *Med Sci Sports Exerc*, 32, pp. 2130–2145.

Anis AH, Stiell IG, Stewart DG, Laupacis A. (1995). Cost-effectiveness analysis of the Ottawa Ankle Rules. *Ann Emerg Med*, 26, pp. 422–428.

Jennings DS, American Dietetic Association. (1995). *Play Hard, Eat Right: A Parent's Guide to Sports Nutrition for Children*. (Wiley, Minneapolis).

Luckstead EF Sr. (2002). Cardiac risk factors and participation guidelines for youth sports. *Pediatr Clin North Am*, 49, pp. 681–707, v.

Luckstead EF Sr. (2002). What is the future potential for pediatric sports medicine? American and international pediatric sport perspectives. *Pediatr Clin North Am*, 49, pp. 857–859, viii.

Lutzenberger W, Elbert T, Rockstroh B, Birbaumer N. (1982). Biofeedback produced slow brain potentials and task performance. *Biol Psychol,* 14, pp. 99–111.

McCambridge TM, Stricker PR, American Academy of Pediatrics Council on Sports Medicine and Fitness. (2008). Strength training by children and adolescents. *Pediatrics*, 121, pp. 835–840.

Metzl JD. (2001). Preparticipation examination of the adolescent athlete: part 1. *Pediatr Rev*, 22, pp. 199–204.

Metzl JD. (2001). Preparticipation examination of the adolescent athlete: part 2. *Pediatr Rev*, 22, pp. 227–239.

Metzl JD, Shookhoff C. (2003). *The Young Athlete: A Sports Doctor's Complete Guide for Parents*. 1st Edn. (Little, Brown and Company, USA).

Norris SL, Lee C, Cea J, Burshteyn D. (1998). Performance enhancement training effects on attention: A case study. *Journal of Neurotherapy*, 3, pp. 19–25.

Perry JJ, Stiell IG. (2006). Impact of clinical decision rules on clinical care of traumatic injuries to the foot and ankle, knee, cervical spine, and head. *Injury,* 37, pp. 1157–1165.

Shepherd R, American Academy of Pediatrics. (1991). Strength training, weight & power lifting, and body building by children and adolescents. *Pediatrics*, 88, pp. 417–418.

Stiell IG, McKnight RD, Greenberg GH, *et al.* (1994). Implementation of the Ottawa ankle rules. *JAMA*, 271, pp. 827–832.

Suggested Websites

American Academy of Pediatrics, Committee on Sports Medicine, policies: http://aappolicy.aappublications.org

International Association of Athletics Federations: http://www.iaaf.org

Chapter 9

Practice Management and New Technologies

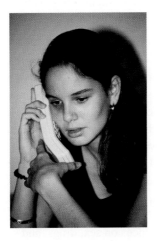

Health is something we do for ourselves, not something that is done to us; a journey rather than a destination; a dynamic, holistic, and purposeful way of living.

— Dr. Elliott Dacher

Overview

Most Adolescent Medicine issues, concerns, risks, behaviors and disorders have remain unchanged since the specialty began in the early 1950s: puberty, sexuality, acne, risk taking, etc. However, current electronic technology, electronic medical records and informational media can now have dramatic impact on adolescent health and wellness.

There are advances in adolescent health screening and assessment, as well as new applications of both common and advanced video and multimedia for health education and promotion. Communicating with media-capable adolescents will be optimally accomplished using technology. Computers and the Internet provide immediate sources of up-to-date information, accessible anywhere. Improved technology and the *need to teach more effectively in less time* has led to the rapid increase in media-based clinical teaching approaches. New office-based communication technology, both on the Internet and via multimedia, will significantly affect adolescent medical practices in the very near future because it will become an expected practice standard, as well as availability, low cost, utility in marketing a practice, better communications with adolescent patients, and the lower cost of media for physician's medical education compared to travel costs. A computer introduces another area of competence that will affect the ability to practice medicine effectively and compete in the Adolescent Medicine marketplace.

Lisa, 17 years old, comes to the clinic and sits at a computer terminal in the waiting room where she completes her automated pre-examination interview. The expert system takes and evaluates medical, health, and behavioral history relevant to the visit. She responds to branching questions for either a health appraisal or the chief complaint of a sick visit, then answers updates for problem areas already in the clinic computer record. She privately watches a clinic information video, and then she sees a video about her assessed chief complaint (acne). She is brought into an examination room where she may finish her computerized interview or health education videos. For a health appraisal, after computerized screening, she watches educational videos on sex, drugs, and safety issues, specific to her screening. The doctor now views his computer which shows him the results of her screening interview, revealing prioritized concerns from the automated assessment. After physical examination, as per the patient's needs, the doctor selects a number of patient education materials on the computer, including a diagnosis-related video on contraception as well as personalized handouts to be printed. Lisa also completes an interactive multimedia game about managing her asthma. The entire office visit was video-recorded (showing her doctor in the examination room with her — including all the counseling, as well as every health education video prescribed) for her to review at home and share with her family; it is also retained for medico-legal documentation in the office. At patient sign-out, the office system burns the entire visit onto video-DVD, prints her future appointment, and all her handouts and patient instructions.

Adolescent Health Informatics

Besides documentation and prescribing, electronic medical records simplify collection and evaluation of data for quality improvement and risk identification within a practice population. Clinical decision support provides prompts to clinicians to improve practice during a visit, and can do proactive quality improvement [Litzelman *et al.*, 1993]. There are comprehensive automated billing processes and procedures for confidential services; a system should use an alternate confidential address for bills associated to a confidential visit and for ancillary services (laboratory, pharmacy), instead of the parents' address [Paperny, 2000].

Adolescent Health Informatics used for Health Care can

- monitor patient and family history.
- screen and manage health problems (acute and chronic illnesses, specific diseases).
- facilitate confidential sexual health care (family planning, STDs, pregnancy).
- detect disease and illnesses (HIV, substance abuse, sexual/physical abuse, violence).
- prescribe electronically.
- provide appropriate anticipatory guidance and health education.

Adolescent Health Informatics used for Practice Management can

- create, download and securely access and store medical records, laboratory and imaging data.
- assure confidentiality and availability of medical records.
- collect and evaluate practice population data.
- submit insurance claims and reportable information.
- schedule appointments.
- accelerate research and dissemination of knowledge.

Adolescent Electronic Medical Records (EMR)

The pressure for clinical quality and patient safety is increasing. EMRs can interconnect clinicians, patients and insurers.

Advantages of Using an EMR

- Increased coding for billing (in some studies: as much as US$40,000 more per MD).
- Captured missing billable items (in some studies: 14% of procedures, 2% of visits).
- Decreased paper chart needs (in some studies: by 90%).
- Improved staff and practitioner morale (in some studies: 4 months after implementation).

- Patients love the technology.
- Quality improvements.
- Improved access to current medical record.
- Prescription legibility.
- Allergy and drug interaction checking.
- Ability to monitor compliance.

EMRs, electronic prescribing, computerized physician order entry, and tele-medicine will dramatically change all aspects of adolescent care. Changes will include paperless offices, electronic "visits" and consultations, home monitoring directly linked to an EMR via the Internet, computer-assisted guidelines monitoring, deci-sion support, and quality reporting — all of which change expectations and standards that also affect medical liability [Paperny, 2009].

Information Managed by an EMR

- Demographics, insurance details, billing and receivables.
- Problem lists, medical history, medication list, allergies.
- Encounter sheets, phone calls/messaging.
- Vital signs, visits: sick and physical examinations.
- Laboratory and X-ray reports.
- Rx refills, school physical forms, vaccination forms.
- Consultant referrals made and notes filed.

Four Categories of Adolescent-Specific Data Required in an EMR

1. Biological
- Vital signs, growth, physical and sexual maturity, and physiologic data.
- Medical history (including hospitalizations, surgeries, medications, allergies).
- Family history (asthma, hyperlipidemia, diabetes).
- Physical examination, normal and abnormal findings.
- Disease-specific findings, diagnoses and therapies.

2. Psychological and Social
- Mental status and cognitive function.
- Affective issues, including depression, suicidal ideation.
- Suicide attempts, self mutilation.
- Abuse (physical, sexual), victimization, bullying.
- Academic achievement and career readiness/performance.
- Legal and economic data, including emancipation and marital status.
- Confidentiality status and confidential contact procedures.

3. Behavioral Risks

- Sexual practices (contraception and high risk sexual behaviors, orientation).
- Safety issues such as firearms, bike helmet and seat belt non-use, driving while intoxicated, riding with intoxicated driver, speeding, racing.
- Exposure to sexual or violent media, exposure to online predators.
- Substance use and abuse.

4. Nutrition and Physical Activity

- Diet (caloric and fat intake), physical activity/caloric expenditure.
- Sports activities and athletics.
- Eating disorders.
- Physical inactivity from media use.

Functionality Provided by a Comprehensive EMR

- Information "at your fingertips".
- Easy documentation and charting.
- Content and tools to improve efficiency, including clinical guidelines/decision support
- Ordering, prescribing (with drug/allergy and drug interaction checking).
- Embedded guidelines to improve quality/efficiency/cost-effectiveness.
- Alerts and reminders.
- Preventive screening and vaccinations.
- Diagnosis/problem list/coding.
- Laboratory/test reporting system/interfaces.
- Practice management/billing system interface.
- Communication and secure messaging.
- Patient access and Internet-based updates by patients.
- Workflow support, including follow-ups and patient education.

Capabilities Facilitated by Use of an EMR

- Clinical and management questions and inquiries.
- Drug recalls management.
- Quality and population disease management (e.g. registries, data queries).
- Outcomes data.
- Case management information.
- Quality and utilization feedback.
- Research (with appropriate safeguards).

Implementation of an EMR creates a significant change. Some physicians will adapt to it more easily than others — learning more quickly to use the system effectively. It may take longer in the beginning, but in the end, the clinician should be more efficient. Physicians' agreement with the statement "An EMR is worth the time and effort required to learn it and use it" increases from 35% at 2 months after EMR implementation to 85% at 4 months [Kaiser Permanente, 2000]. The effective use of computers leverages integrated delivery.

What to Expect from an Established EMR

- Significantly increased workflow — increased patient load via enhanced efficiency.
- Reduced patient-management time.
- Reduced errors — and litigation.
- Augmented bottom line — increased income later, after initial investment.
- Better patient service — they will like it.

Time and Effort of Implementation and Use of an EMR is Offset by

- readily available medical information, handouts, lab reports, and radiograph readings.
- reduction in errors and litigation from thorough documentation/templates used for visit notes.
- workflow efficiency.
- legible prescriptions: reduction in incoming calls from pharmacists.
- patient satisfaction: patients appreciate a high-tech system, clear patient handouts, prescriptions, and information sheets.

When children reach the age to consent to specific confidential services (varies by jurisdiction), laws restrict online proxy access to patient health information. Parents and guardians then lose their access to an adolescent's record (in the absence of incompetence certification). Direct access by teens is impacted by laws such as the United States Children's Online Privacy Protection Act, which requires "verifiable parental consent" for online transactions (i.e. direct access) for children under the age of 13. Unanticipated disclosures of confidential adolescent visits sometimes result from unexpected electronic business/insurance notifications of care [Paperny, 2009].

> To determine if he is updated on chlamydia STD screening levels for his patients, the doctor uses the office medical record computer system to evaluate his population of high risk adolescents by selecting ages 13–25. Then he selects the subgroup that has had any of these findings suggesting sexual experience: 1. Had a prior chlamydia, gonorrhea or pregnancy test, or 2. Had a prescription for oral

contraceptive, or 3. Received Depo-Provera, or 4. Received emergency contraception) and had no chlamydia test in the past 1 year. He then reviews each chart and notifies each patient who is due for a screening test by using a predetermined confidential method selected by the patient — often a private cell phone, sometimes secure email messaging, but almost never a letter to the home.

Communications with Adolescent Patients

Adolescents are comfortable with communication tools, and these devices can facilitate health care. Most messaging (cell phone texting, email) between a clinic and adolescents creates neither an office visit charge nor confidential billing issues. Short messaging service (SMS) is useful since adolescent patients can receive or send a message of up to 160 characters to a cell phone or personal digital assistant (PDA). Messaging can answer confidential clinical questions and provide appointment reminders. Electronic communication tools and text messaging on cell phones as well as email or secure electronic messaging are ideal for adolescent patients, but "confidential" text messages to cellphones are not secure as there is usually no password protection.

Texting is a health tool for adolescents and gives them a sense of autonomy [Chen, 2009; www.texting4health.org]. It improves compliance and outcomes among transplant patients and those with other chronic diseases. CareSpeak, a program for liver transplant patients, used text messages to remind patients to take their medications, and patients were more likely to take their medications and experienced less rejection episodes. Sweet Talk, a text-messaging support system enhances self-efficacy, facilitates insulin therapy, and improves glycemic control in adolescent patients with type 1 diabetes [Franklin *et al.*, 2003; Krishna and Boren, 2008]. SMS and multimedia message service (MMS) obesity management improved weight loss in a study group that received daily messages compared to the control group [Patrick *et al.*, 2009]. Mobile phone-based motivation and action support systems have been shown to increase and maintain levels of physical activity, with more loss of body fat and true increase in moderate physical activity than controls [Haapala *et al.*, 2009].

A message can include a photograph of the exact pill to take, reminders for medication refills, creating a text message support group, and sending patients positive feedback and motivational messages from physicians and other members of the care management team, for almost any chronic disease, and with anyone who needs reminders. Such communications can help enhance the relationship between adolescent patients and their clinicians.

Mobile technology is used by almost all adolescents worldwide now, with cell phones, smartphones and hybrids capable of photo and text messaging, MP3 (music and sound), video, photo camera and video camera, calendar reminders, alarms, and Internet service with built-in wireless broadband. Podcasts are a new form of sharing audio, video and other health education information through multimedia message services (MMS).

Email with Adolescent Patients

Over 75% of patients say patient email messaging improves access to their providers. E-visits are more time-efficient than office visits (for both MD and patients) and returning patients' phone calls [Leiderman, Morefield, 2003; Gerstle, 2004]. However, emails are like telephone calls; although they are usually patient-password protected, they are not encrypted or authenticated, and they may breach privacy by using employer email. They have no charge capture function, no template or medical records features, and are usually not "safety-proofed" for healthcare. The effective and convenient use of personal email with adolescents requires pre-planning with office policies in place, but secure messaging is available from several Internet services (that collect a small fee).

Anatomy of an Email Message
- Address: user@host (case-independent, no spaces).
- Subject line (Jimmy MR#445566 re: acne).
- Message body (Text: typed or copied).
- E-signature.
- Attachments (describe all attachments).

Email Acceptable Uses
- Prescription refills.
- Documentation requests, forms.
- General, non-urgent questions.
- Laboratory results (especially if confidential).
- Routine follow-up/chronic disease management, i.e. diabetes mellitus.
- Confidential/sensitive questions (i.e. bleeding on Depo-Provera).
- Appointment reminders (vs calls, especially confidential).

Email Communication Guidelines
- Establish turnaround time: often 2–4 days if not on vacation.
- Disclose privacy issues: who sees messages when the doctor is away.
- Establish acceptable uses and guidelines for sensitive matters.

- Content of the Subject line should indicate type of message.
- Require patient ID: MR# and/or birth date in Subject line or body of message.
- Auto-reply & out of office responses: "Email received; expect answer in a few days," "Away from office until April 9. Call 432-0000 for assistance."
- Print and put in paper chart, or copy into EMR.
- Request acknowledgment from patients.
- Maintain a mailing list of patients — use blind copying feature (bcc).

Email Administrative and Legal Guidelines

- Put your email policies and rules in writing (sign Informed Consent?).
- Patient must agree to terms of your communication guidelines, including NO forwarding, marketing, or sharing doctor's email address.
- Terms for "escalation" to telephone.
- Describe security protocols — and lack thereof (waive encryption).
- Disclaimer for equipment failures.
- Data backup policy and procedure, both short term and long term.

The most important part of the physician's email is the signature [Paperny, 2006]. Automatically append it to every outgoing message. Keep it short (5–7 lines).

Elements Required in an Email Signature

- Doctor's Name, relevant degrees
- Address, telephone and fax numbers
- Best email address used for *patients only*
- Disclaimers and other standard information: "In case of emergency…," "This is not medical advice.", "This is not my legal signature."

Internet Patient Communications and the Clinician's Website

Numerous services offer different functionality for clinical practice websites. Many physicians create their own. The site can link to Internet sites used by adolescents to obtain health education and information. We know three-quarters of all adolescents use the Internet for health education information, and two-thirds use it for health information for school-related projects [Borzekowski, 2001].

Useful Internet Sites to Link with Reliable Health Information

- TeenGrowth.com
- TeensHealth.org
- GoAskAlice.columbia.edu
- nida.nih.gov

- Teen-Matters.com
- AdolescentHealth.org

The functionality of an office/clinic website can include the personal health record (PHR). 70% of Internet users want an online PHR to store immunization results, track medications, look up test results, and transfer medical histories to new health care providers. Other patient communications files can be downloaded from the physician's website, or these media can be shared in the office. Adolescents can take home files on an iPod/MP3 player or USB memory stick, or simply beam them to their cellphone.

Useful File Types to Share with Adolescents
- .doc — document (Word processor) files, handouts, etc.
- .txt — document (text) files (easy to email too!)
- .jpg — photo files (email and doctor's website)
- .mp3 — audio files (doctor's website: podcasts)
- .mpg — video files (examination room video, MPEG-1)

Tele-Medicine

SMS was used to send patient-specific recommendations to a group of patients with diabetes after they sent in daily reports on glucose, diet, and exercise to the clinician; those patients had decreased HBA1c measurements [Cole-Lewis and Kershaw, 2010]. Care for Asthma via Mobile Phone (CAMP) program was developed in Taiwan using mobile phones to give patient-specific feedback on their peak flow meter results and demonstrated a significant benefit in improving the compliance with medications in asthma.

Remote video now enables providers to interview, assess, and counsel adolescents as if they were present in the office or clinic. Patients can also send photographs to clinicians by email, and communicate using webcams and live video on the Internet. Potentially, for an adolescent at home, it will be possible to "visit" the doctor and get a video-consult by using an in-home digital still-camera or live-action video. It allows the clinician to "see" the patient, to make therapeutic recommendations, and deliver advice and health education, saving both the adolescent and the clinician time and expense [Tidwell, 1998]. A patient can be emailed health education media described above. Successes seen in dermatology and other specialties relate to the relative costs of getting patients in to see specialists.

Medical Education Technology

Multimedia message service (MMS) has been used for clinical care purposes, but also more recently for academic and medical educational purposes; ReachMD has made continuing medical education credits available as podcasts (www.reachmd.com). A number of professional organizations now offer continuing medical education credits for viewing videocasts of their professional conferences. Medical students have been given PDAs with required reading material for the clinical rotations. Nursing educators have used PDAs to enhance students' pharmacological and clinical knowledge; those using the PDAs had increases in their scores in pharmacological and clinical knowledge, twice the increases of a control group. PDAs enhance undergraduate clinical nursing education at National University of Singapore with wireless-enabled PDAs.

Computerized Adolescent Health Screening and Assessment

In order to deliver more cost-effective services to adolescents, creative use of automation can expand the capacity of the clinic or office [Elster, 1993]. Allied health professionals and paraprofessionals, along with use of educational technology, can expand our capacity to deliver a fuller range of services to the many adolescents at-risk [Paperny, Hedberg, 1999]. Early detection and risk assessment with personalized interventions are essential to manage adolescent health issues. Computer-assisted health evaluation of an adolescent's needs and problems can enhance the timeliness and reliability of health care. Technology that allows health providers to easily access useful behavioral and medical information helps health providers make sounder medical decisions, facilitates personalized advice and improves case management.

The personal health interview and counseling can be simulated by expert interactive software, which uses complex rule-based algorithms for branching and decision making [Rathbun, 1993]. Automated interview assessments accomplish a health evaluation by proceeding logically in the history-taking format of a trained clinician. Complex relational algorithms and built-in clinical logic validations assess health risks and behaviors, while the branching of questions depends on the adolescent's responses which also control educational feedback to be administered. Such a rule-based, interactive program accomplishes a directed history based on screening questions and previous answers. Internal cross-validation of responses for consistency and the opportunity to backtrack to clarify answers maximizes specificity of the interview. An automated interview minimizes interpersonal barriers such as avoidance, discomfort, denial and confidentiality concerns. Such a screening interview-assessment can be done by telephone automation (press a number or speak a response), by Internet, or on a personal computer or network terminal.

Uses of Screening and Educational Technology for Adolescent Health Promotion
- Screening for risk intervention and case management (drug or alcohol use, sexual activity).

- Evaluation of preventive care needs and anticipatory guidance.
- Assessment for necessary illness-detection and testing (STD risk, hepatitis-B risk).
- Provide rule-based or artificial-intelligence-based problem list support.
- Designate patient-need-specific multimedia and health education.

Both screening questionnaires [Schubiner *et al.*, 1994] and computerized health assessments [Webb *et al.*, 1999] have helped to improve services for adolescents at risk. Technology can also help adolescents evaluate the consequences of their health behavior choices. Medical [Grossman, 1971], psychosocial [Greist, 1973] and behavioral histories [Space, 1981] are easily obtained, and adolescents indicate that they do prefer interactive computer interviews [Slack, 1971] and training programs [Fisher *et al.*, 1977] on most sensitive topics rather than direct human interventions. Adolescents freely reveal sensitive information to computers. Researchers at UCSF Adolescent Clinic [Millstein and Irwin, 1983] interviewed 108 adolescent girls about sexual behavior, and compared a mainframe computer program, a self-administered questionnaire, and a face-to-face interview. Adolescents preferred the computer interview method and were more comfortable with the computer, finding it "private", "easy", "fun", and "interesting".

Educational feedback can be generated from computerized health history questions when associations between responses are provided by an expert system. The resulting personalized feedback can facilitate higher-level interventions that would usually be too time-consuming and impractical to attain in many clinical settings.

Capabilities of Expert Interview Software

- Obtain a thorough health and behavioral history.
- Identify and prioritize problem areas and health needs.
- Provide appropriate health advice and local referrals, and age-specific anticipatory guidance.
- Administer pertinent, succinct health education videos.
- Dispense understandable customized take-home materials.
- Provide assessment data and problem list for clinician's use.

An adolescent-based study of such computer-assisted self interview (CASI) with feedback algorithms showed the comparison between 265 anonymous computer users and a matched group of 294 users who were pre-directed to share a printout of their responses to sensitive questions with a clinician [Paperny, 1990]. Sensitive questions included information on sexual behavior, interest in contraceptive information, and adjustment/emotional issues. Both the two computer groups (anonymous vs to be shared) were comparable in sensitivity and were both better in detecting sensitive issues than the matched written questionnaire (to be shared) group of 240. This suggested superiority of the computer over the written questionnaire for detecting sensitive issues. Verbally expressing risk behaviors and anticipated clinician disapproval were the main barriers, but the computer was perceived as anonymous and non-judgmental.

CASI assessments of adolescent opinion and self-report on the computer interview process [Paperny, 1997] included 4,266 first-time users (3,276 adolescents in medical clinic settings, 640 in public health fair settings, and 288 in detention or youth corrections facility; ages 13–19, mean 15.5 years, 54% female). Interview process evaluation responses were given before automated feedback was printed for the adolescent and reflect the questioning process by the computer. To the question "How honest and accurate have you been with me on these questions?", 85% of the adolescents responded that they were totally honest and accurate, 8% that they were not completely honest, 5% that they could not understand some of it, and 2% that they were pretty inaccurate. The computer method was preferred by 89%, while only 5% preferred a personal interview, and 6% a paper-based questionnaire. When asked "How did you like talking to the computer?", 85% responded positively, 12% neutral, and 3% negatively. Data were collected on risk behaviors and revealed 10% of males and 15% of females had attempted suicide. Nearly half of the adolescents were sexually experienced, and 16% of females had a significant risk of being pregnant based on responses. For a subgroup of 200 adolescents, 97% responded they "told the computer their real and true information", 96% felt "the computer asked good questions", 95% reported that they "read the printout", and 97% felt "the content made good sense to them".

The most important conclusion these studies suggest is that *divulging* of sensitive information is not the problem — indeed adolescents want to — but the "non-personal" *method* of obtaining it by computer protects them from embarrassment and judgmentalism. Computer-assisted assessment of health needs and risks is thorough, accurate, painless, easy, and saves interviewer time.

Computer-Assisted Health Promotion and Adolescent Preventive Services

Every opportunity should be used to identify high-risk adolescents and also to administer and reinforce health promotion messages. To optimize clinical outcomes, we need to offer adolescents health education using the most familiar media — television, video, and computers. We normally speak to adolescents to communicate medical advice, but understanding, acceptance, assimilation and retention of verbal advice varies widely, as does compliance with health recommendations [Bartlett, 1984]. The usual written instructions and printed brochures are often provided and discarded, but we can now use technology which constitutes far more acceptable and effective patient education. Routine anticipatory health guidance should be provided by a variety of methods and media (e.g. patient groups, audio-visual materials and interactive multimedia, and referral to trusted Internet sites) [Rosen *et al.*, 1997]. Because cognitive services and health education are time-intensive, health providers and clinics should consider information technology and utilization of specialized paraprofessional manpower for producing improved yet cost-effective clinical outcomes. Appropriate combinations of allied health personnel, health educators, as well as peer counselors working with screening and educational information technology offer a potent intervention approach to adolescent health promotion in various settings [Paperny, Hedberg, 1999].

Currently, the Youth Health Program software (by HealthMediaCorp.com) provides feedback including interactive, personalized multimedia presentations followed by printed information with specific health advice and referrals to health resources. The program conserves professional time when the clinician is given the printed problem list based on the adolescent's interview responses. It has been used in clinics, schools, community agencies and other settings, as part of health evaluation visits with clinicians and as a "stand-alone" assessment and educational tool at kiosks, health fairs, and education centers (self-service, requiring no supervision). The software internally validates responses for consistency with prior screening responses and reconfirms crucial branch point questions, maximizing specificity (see Appendix). The interactive, multimedia presentations are culturally diverse; each youth using the program, after answering questions about his/her gender and racial background, will have assessment questions and educational materials delivered by videos of culturally-similar youths (in English or Spanish), maximizing rapport and credibility. Automated health education and age-specific anticipatory guidance is prioritized, confidential, credible, creates more retention, and saves educator time.

> *Youth Health Program software — A comprehensive program for adolescent health appraisal and education. Time saving and reliable. Identifies health-risk behaviors and their seriousness more accurately than a face-to-face interview.*
>
> — Adele Hofmann MD

Health Promotion and Health Education Using Video, DVD, Multimedia

Since clinicians give guidance by repeating daily the same standardized health information to adolescents, there is increasing demand to use video and multimedia as enhancements to the spoken and printed word. Appropriate anticipatory and routine health guidance may be provided by a variety of information technology and media within the clinic setting (video, computer-based interactive multimedia, and/or Internet sites) [Rosen *et al.*, 1997]. Video-enhanced health education may be one of the best ways to facilitate standardized communication that has proven effective with adolescents. Surveys suggest that patient education videos are desired by both clinicians and patients in over 80% of office visits [Paperny, Zurhellen, *et al.*, 1999].

Current, easy-to-use storage media (CD-ROM & DVD) allow dissemination of huge amounts of information: audio, video, animation, and motion graphics to educate patients both in the office or clinic and at home. There are four major requirements of effective health education video: understandable scripting, succinct presentations, use effectiveness with results evaluation, and ease of administration. Routine video use in clinical settings is usually limited by a number of obstacles: the non-standard paradigm, patient flow/space limitations, limited videos available, most existing videos are long, inefficient and have not been target-population tested for effect, lack simple layman's language to ensure comprehension, and do not use "television-quality production techniques" to hold viewer attention. For practical office use, a video topic must be short and powerfully presented (i.e. like MTV commercials).

Quality Videos

1. have a concise 1–3 minute format that holds patients' attention and does not obstruct examination rooms and patient flow.
2. are succinct vignettes that emphasize main points and priority advice.
3. use no talking heads.
4. make main points by voice-over spoken messages.
5. use warm close-ups, good lighting, and frequent scene changes (every 4 seconds).
6. have camera angles which avoid a recognizable doctor — a custom-produced look.
7. have meticulous script wording which is understandable, non-technical, universal, and avoids controversy and bias.

The most valuable use of health education videos is to teach the basics and allow more advanced use of professional or educator time to evaluate understanding and readiness for behavior change. There is a trend toward more efficient use of physician time while also meeting more educational standards and requirements. Health education video technology can be the best tool to teach standard health care basics, and it allows precise medical record documentation of information provided (video script content).

Direct video reinforcement of a clinician's advice is a useful adjunct to enhance patient understanding, retention, and compliance [Paperny, 1992]. More focus and attention is often given to television screens than to actual persons: Studies show jurors' attention is more focused when court proceedings are watched on a remote television rather than in person in a courtroom. A video efficacy study [Paperny, 1994] compared adolescent video watchers to handout readers: 595 anonymous adolescents at outpatient physical exams were randomly divided into three matched groups — Group 1: computer-administered videos, Group 2: computer-dispensed handouts (identical to the video scripts) which were actually read, and Group 3: (controls) used computer but received no handouts or videos. Before and after computer use, knowledge items on the content of each video script about sex and smoking were measured on the three groups. Both media groups showed significantly greater knowledge gains than the control group, but *video* watchers had 57% more knowledge improvements than *handout* readers.

Another study showed compliance with medical treatment and follow-up improved by 50% when medical advice was followed by video viewing [Paperny DM, 1991]. Compliance was 65% when the patient was counseled by the physician alone, 60% when counseled by the physician and given a handout, and 90% when counseling by the physician was followed by video viewing. Video can enable clinicians to demonstrate home management techniques, and it can validate medical advice for skeptical adolescents and dramatize consequences that they should anticipate from high risk health choices [Gagliano, 1988]. When videos are to be used for health education, one must be aware of criteria for evaluation of patient education video when incorporating and using them in the clinical setting.

Administration of Video in Medical Settings

Video and television is ubiquitous for adolescents worldwide. In the busy medical setting, it is not practical to use cumbersome videotapes which require rewinding and searching for topics and eventually wear out. Current digital compact videodisks eliminate these problems. The format called video-CD is simpler than DVD, and the video-CD video files (MPEG-1) can be shown on any examination room computer terminal used for CASI or as an examination room EMR.

It has been impractical for busy emergency rooms caring for adolescents to routinely use educational videos because of high patient flow. Asthma is a common condition affecting many adolescents with poor self-management skills. An emergency room (ER) demonstration project [Boychuck *et al.*, 2006] used immediate asthma training with an interactive, branching DVD (by HealthMediaCorp.com) to teach asthma care skills, often while receiving nebulizer treatment. Headphones for patients were used with succinct presentations designed to not limit patient flow. Physicians prescribed relevant DVD video selections on preprinted Asthma-Video-Rx forms, and ER staff administered each prescribed video. The Asthma Care DVD branched through 19 age-specific topics. Testing and follow-up showed that patient compliance and asthma care skills were enhanced by supplementing ER treatments with video health education.

Multimedia message services (MMS) support the role of mobile portable technology, including direct downloads of videocasts to personal digital assistants (PDAs), in both patient education and in improving clinical outcomes. Oral health of adolescents worldwide is generally poor, and such technology has been used to improve the oral health of people with mild to moderate intellectual disabilities. A set of studies [Brock, Smith, 2007; Smith, Brock *et al.*, 2003; Smith, Rublein *et al.*, 2003] analyzed the role of educational videos on PDAs for patients with human immunodeficiency virus; they demonstrated a significant ($p < 0.05$) improvement in medication adherence as well as knowledge of disease and medications.

Computer-Assisted Instruction (CAI) Games

Experiential computer programs and games can facilitate mature, informed decision making by adolescents who need not suffer the embarrassment or actual consequences of poor health choices. CAI influences patient attitudes, beliefs, feelings and knowledge, even on sensitive health subjects [Bosworth *et al.*, 1983]. Adolescents enjoy animated-action, color computer games and training software, which capture and hold attention by using problem-solving situations, simulations, and scenarios. Game-format CAI algorithms are powerful, health education tools which are interactive/responsive, provide information, and simulate outcomes creating the impact of reality. Risk-taking and "reality testing" by adolescents may be modified by automated choice assessment in combination with directed educational feedback, giving them better decision making information. Adolescents actively explore health alternatives and outcomes, then experience consequences of their choices. Interactive educational games can modify adolescent health behaviors by sharing knowledge, correcting misconceptions, and allowing adolescents to practice desired behaviors and appropriate decision making skills. They have also been shown to reduce counseling time and facilitate acceptance and retention of critical health concepts [Krishna, 1997].

Two CAI games for preventing adolescent pregnancy and parenting demonstrated improvements in attitudes, beliefs, feelings, and knowledge on these sensitive subjects [Paperny, Starn, 1989]. Both games resulted in statistically significant improvements in user groups when compared with controls. A study [Timpka *et al.*, 2004] evaluating computer game designs found that playing educational games was mainly motivated by the challenges and competition represented in the gaming scripts.

Interactive Patient Health Education Multimedia

Interactive multimedia is defined as the use of a software program to control various media output and feedback so that the branching and decision making of the process is continually dependent on the trainee's choices or responses. Many medical schools and the world's largest companies use interactive video and multimedia for training and education because they produce strong reinforcement that helps trainees learn twice as fast as standard instruction. Interactive health education multimedia offers the combination of visual presentation with audio explanation, making information quickly and easily understandable and keeps an adolescent's attention focused. Immediate feedback provides continual, personalized reinforcement of material and is highly motivating. Over three dozen studies show such interactive technology reduces learning time by 50% and improves retention of material by more than 25% [Howsie, 1987; Schwier, 1987]. Mastery of content occurs by quickly finishing strength areas and concentrating on areas of weakness. It does not require any clinician time, and it can be delivered privately and consistently, 24 hours a day without interpersonal performance stress or embarrassment. It can be used in the office or clinic, verbally reinforced before completion of a visit, and then reviewed at home.

Evaluation Criteria for Health Video and Multimedia

- Length of presentation and administration plans.
- Video production techniques used (quality).
- Instructional formats used: lecture, voice-over, demonstration, testimonials.
- Accuracy of information and script content.
- Timelessness: content not soon out of date — appearance and attire (fashion).
- Formal evaluation documentation: understandability, acceptability, learning — pre-post testing.

There are four general criteria for evaluating and implementing clinical software programs: features, content, capabilities, and customizability.

Considerations for Selecting and Implementing Adolescent Health Education Hardware, Software, Video and Multimedia for use in the clinic setting

- Cost (hardware and software) and office space requirements.
- Staffing and administrative, computer technical support requirement.
- Accessibility, usability and appropriateness for use by adolescents.
- Hardware/software requirements: office system vs a dedicated system.
- Content quality and accuracy.
- Patient benefits and impact on health outcomes.

[from Paperny, Zurhellen, *et al.*, 1999]

Emerging Technologies and Future Trends

Server networks allow integration of health screening and education materials with a total information system and an electronic medical record. Adolescent informatics integration [Zurhellen, 1995] includes medical providers, hospitals, laboratories, specialists, video-consultative services, medical information networks, health education vendors, e-mail services, and Internet services. With improved integration, an amazing array of medical and health information technology will interact seamlessly to create an efficient and convenient health screening and education system previously unknown in health care.

The plethora of modes of sharing information in many formats is perfect for well-wired adolescent patients. Advertisers pay for the attention of adolescents and young adults — to have their products in the eye or ear for only a moment. *Incentives* to adolescents for health education and promotion can facilitate attention paid to repetitive positive health messages. Repetitive violent and negative messages in television, music, and computer games can be replaced by positive content. Studies show that monetary incentives affect adolescent behavior [Stevens-Simon *et al.*, 1997]. They facilitate participation in health education programs and promote peer-support group attendance. Therefore, offering "web credits" to youths' electronic accounts could promote attention to positive health messages. Health screening and feedback advice may be done by kiosks (for coupons and other incentives) at fast food restaurants and shopping malls where adolescents spend their time.

Many adolescents' reasons for medical visits are psychosomatic or cognitive issues, therefore it will benefit adolescents to provide assertiveness skills, personal empowerment tools, stress management techniques, and even subconscious suggestions for positive health. Technology is now able to interface the subconscious mind with creative thinking, modeling and health-enhancing messages using various media including music, video, and worldwide participation Internet games. Even all-night-sleep affirmations for health and well-being could potentially promote positive health attitudes and choices. Technology such as biofeedback (including brainwave biofeedback) can also interface the body and mind. Such internal balance and centering techniques can facilitate higher brain functions and health.

The human body is an 80% water-based crystalloid-protein emulsion which may hold information and consciousness on levels of which we remain unaware. Dr. Emoto's experiments with water [Emoto, 2004; Radin *et al.*, 2006] suggest that water alone can hold information; a tissue example is that heart transplant patients sometimes manifest verifiable memories belonging to their donor. This has implications for health and new ways of learning. The multifunction Internet cellphones that keep adolescents "connected to the grid" will eventually be miniaturized to the size of chips which can be implanted near the ears to provide communication and Internet services (including stereo music) on demand.

When technology is used to positively promote healthy choices and attitudes, our technologically advanced adolescents will engage useful health information on many levels (vs the continual feed of negative information such as disease-based television commercials, violent television programming, negative rap music, etc.). When adolescents attend to and accept information that empowers them to make optimal personal health and well-being choices, this *proactive approach* will cost society far less than the reactive approach and palliative damage control. What better use of technology than to screen for those health and well-being attitudes and behaviors which are counterproductive, and reframe them toward the positive. It is important that the content of media information provided to youth possess content which enhances health and well-being [Strasburger, 2006]. Education is the imparting of useful and creative ideas to those who make room for them. The application of new, yet common, technologies will facilitate this progress in Adolescent Medicine and Health Promotion.

Suggested Readings and Bibliography

Alur P, Cirelli J, Goodstein M, Bell T, Liss J. (2009). Role of handheld PCs in disease comprehension by parents in the NICU. Poster presentation at PAS-SPR conference, May 2009. (Baltimore, MD).

American Academy of Pediatrics, Task Force on Medical Informatics, Section on Computers and Other Technologies (incl. David Paperny MD), Committee on Practice and Ambulatory Medicine. (1996). Safeguards needed in transfer of patient data. *Pediatrics*, 98, pp. 984–986.

Bartlett EE. (1984). Effective approaches to patient education for the busy pediatrician. *Pediatrics*, 74(Suppl), pp. 920–923.

Borzekowski DL, Rickert VI. (2001). Adolescent cybersurfing for health information: a new resource that crosses barriers. *Arch Pediatr Adolesc Med*, 155, pp. 813–817.

Bosworth K, Gustafson D, Hawkins R, Chewning B, Day T. (1983). Adolescents, health education and computers: The Body Awareness Resource Network (BARN). *Health Educ*, 14, pp. 58–60.

Boychuk R, DeMesa C, Kiyabu K, *et al.* (2006). Change in approach and delivery of medical care in children with asthma: results from a multicenter emergency department educational asthma management program. *Pediatrics*, 117, pp. S145–S151; and Managing Pediatric Asthma: Emergency Department Demonstration Program, Robert Wood Johnson Grant Reference ID#047512, "The Asthma Care DVD–An Interactive DVD to Teach Asthma Care Skills" by HealthMedia Corp., Lafayette, Colorado.

Brock TP, Smith SR. (2007). Using digital videos displayed on personal digital assistants (PDAs) to enhance patient education in clinical settings. *Int J Med Inform*, 76, pp. 829–835.

Bynum AB, Cranford CO, Irwin CA, Denny GS. (2003). Participant satisfaction in an adult telehealth education program using interactive compressed video delivery methods in rural Arkansas. *J Rural Health*. 19, pp. 218–222.

Chen M. (1983). How effective are microcomputer-based programs for health education: a prospective view. *Health Educ*, 14, pp. 88–89.

Chen P. (2009). Texting as a Health Tool for Teenagers. *New York Times* (Published: November 5).

Cole-Lewis H, Kershaw T. (2010). Text Messaging as a tool for behavior change in disease prevention and management. *Epidemiol Rev*, 32, pp. 56–69.

Elster AB. (1993). Confronting the crisis in adolescent health: visions for change. *J Adolesc Health*, 14, pp. 505–508.

Emoto M. (2004). Healing with water. *J Altern Complement Med*, 10, pp. 19–21.

Fisher LA, Johnson T, Porters D, *et al.* (1977). Collection of a clean voided urine specimen: a comparison among spoken, written, and computer-based instructions. *Am J Public Health*, 67, pp. 640–644.

Franklin V, Waller A, Pagliari C, Greene S. (2003). "Sweet Talk": text messaging support for intensive insulin therapy for young people with diabetes. *Diabetes Technol Ther*, 5, pp. 991–996.

Gagliano M. (1988). A literature review on the efficacy of video in patient education. *J Med Educ*, 63, pp. 785–792.

Gerstle R and AAP Task Force on Medical Informatics. (2004). E-mail communication between pediatricians and their patients. *Pediatrics*, 114, pp. 317–321.

Greist J. (1973). A computer interview for suicide risk prediction. *Am J Psychiatry*, 130, p. 1327.

Grossman S. (1971). Evaluation of computer acquired patient histories. *JAMA*, 215, p. 1286.

Haapala I, Barengo NC, Biggs S, Surakka L, Manninen P. (2009). Weight loss by mobile phone: a 1-year effectiveness study. *Public Health Nutr*, 12, pp. 2382–2391.

Havel RD, Wright MP. (1997). Automated interviewing for hepatitis B risk assessment and vaccination referral. *Am J Prev Med*, 13, pp. 392–395.

Howsie P. (1987). Adopting interactive videodisc technology for education. *Educ Technology*, July, pp. 5–10.

Kaiser Permanente Hawaii. (2000). Clinical Information System — Provider and Operational Forum, "Common Themes", May 24–25.

Krishna S, Boren SA. (2008). Diabetes self-management care via cell phone: a systematic review. *J Diabetes Sci Technol*, 2, pp. 509–517.

Krishna S. (1997). Clinical trials of interactive computerized patient education: implications for family practice. *J Fam Pract*, 45, pp. 25–33.

Liederman E, Morefield C. (2003). Web messaging: a new tool for patient-physician communication. *J Am Med Inform Assoc*, 10, pp. 260–270.

Litzelman DK, Dittus RS, Miler ME, *et al.* (1993). Requiring physicians to respond to computerized reminders improves their compliance with preventive care protocols. *J Gen Intern Med*, 8, pp. 311–317.

Mangunkusumo R, Moorman P, Van Den Berg-de Ruiter A, *et al.* (2005). Internet-administered adolescent health questionnaires compared with paper version in a randomized study *J Adolesc Health*, 36, p. 70.

Marco CA, Larkin GL. (2003). Public education regarding resuscitation: effects of a multimedia intervention. *Ann Emerg Med*, 42, pp. 256–260.

Millstein S, Irwin C. (1983). Acceptability of computer-acquired sexual histories in adolescent girls. *J Pediatr*, 103, pp. 815–819.

Paperny DM, Aono JY, Lehman RM, *et al*. (1988). Computer-assisted detection, evaluation, and referral of sexually abused adolescents. *J Adolesc Health Care*, 9, p. 260.

Paperny DM, Starn JR. (1989). Adolescent pregnancy prevention by health education computer games: computer-assisted instruction of knowledge and attitudes. *Pediatrics*, 83, pp. 742–752.

Paperny DM, Aono JY, Lehman RM, *et al*. (1990). Computer-assisted detection and intervention in adolescent high-risk health behaviors. *J Pediatr*, 116, pp. 456–462.

Paperny DM. (1991). HMO innovations. Video-enhanced medical advice. *HMO Pract*, 5, pp. 212–213.

Paperny D. (1991). Computers and Patient Education. *Computers for the Practicing Pediatrician*. 2nd Edn. (American Academy of Pediatrics, Illinois).

Paperny DM. (1992). Pediatric medical advice enhanced with use of video. *Am J Dis Child*, 146, pp. 785–786.

Paperny DM. (1994). Automated adolescent preventative services using computer-assisted video multimedia. *J Adolesc Health*, 15, p. 66.

Paperny D. (1995). Patient Education Computers, Videos and Multimedia. *Computers for the Practicing Pediatrician*. 3rd Edn. (American Academy of Pediatrics, Illinois).

Paperny DM. (1997). Computerized health assessment and education for adolescent HIV and STD prevention in health care settings and schools. *Health Educ Behav*, 24, pp. 54–70.

Paperny DM. (2000). Computers and information technology: implications for the 21st century. *Adolesc Med*, 11, pp. 183–202.

Paperny D. (2006). *Communicating With Your Teen Patients by E-Mail: It's Easy!* Society for Adolescent Medicine annual meeting: Hot Topics plenary session, March 24, 2006.

Paperny D. (2007). Office-based computerized risk-assessment and health education systems. *Adolesc Med State Art Rev*, 18, pp. 256–270.

Paperny D. (2009). Special health information needs of adolescent care. In: Lehmann C, Kim GR, Johnson KB (eds), *Pediatric Informatics: Computer Applications in Child Health*, pp. 43–53 (Springer, NY).

Paperny D. (2009). Privacy Issues. In: Lehmann C, Kim GR, Johnson KB (eds), *Pediatric Informatics: Computer Applications in Child Health*, pp. 303–310 (Springer, NY).

Paperny D. (2010). Computers, technology and the Internet. In: *Textbook of Adolescent Health Care*. (in press 2010). (American Academy of Pediatrics, Elk Grove Village).

Paperny D, Hedberg V. (1999). Computer-assisted health counselor visits: A low-cost model for comprehensive adolescent preventive services. *Arch Pediatr Adolesc Med*, 153, pp. 63–67.

Paperny D, Zurhellen W, *et al*. (1999). "W415: Advanced Clinical Computing Strategies." American Academy of Pediatrics Annual Meeting, 6-hour Workshop sponsored by Section on Computers & Other Technologies. October 12, Washington D.C.

Parker-Pope T. (2009). Texting for Better Health. *New York Times*. Available form: http://well.blog.nytimes.com/2009/11/05/texting-for-better-health

Patrick K, Raab F, Adams MA, *et al*. (2009). A text message-based intervention for weight loss: randomized controlled trial. *J Med Internet Res*, 11, p. e1.

Radin D, Hayssen G, Emoto M, Kizu T. (2006). Double-blind test of the effects of distant intention on water crystal formation. *Explore* (*NY*), 2, pp. 408–411.

Rathbun J. (1993). Development of a computerized alcohol screening instrument for the university community. *J Am Coll Health*, 42, pp. 33–36.

Robinson JS, Schwartz ML, Magwene KS, *et al.* (1989). The impact of fever health education on clinic utilization. *Am J Dis Child*, 143, pp. 698–704.

Rosen D, Elster A, Hedberg V, Paperny D. (1997). Clinical preventive services for adolescents: position paper of the Society for Adolescent Medicine. *J Adolesc Health*, 21, pp. 203–214.

Schubiner H, Tzelepis A, Wright K, *et al.* (1994). The clinical utility of the Safe Times Questionnaire. *J Adolesc Health*, 15, pp. 374–382.

Swartz LH, Noell JW, Schroeder SW, Ary DV. (2006). A randomized control study of a fully automated Internet based smoking cessation programe. *Tob Control*, 15. pp. 7–12.

Schwier R. (1987). *Interactive Video*. (Educational Technology Publications, Englewood Cliffs).

Slack WV. (1971). Computer-based interviewing system dealing with nonverbal behavior as well as keyboard responses. *Science*, 171, pp. 84–87.

Smith SR, Brock TP, Howarth SM. (2005). Use of personal digital assistants to deliver education about adherence to antiretroviral medications. *J Am Pharm Assoc*, 45, pp. 625–628.

Smith SR, Rublein JC, Marcus C, *et al.* (2003). A medication self-management program to improve adherence to HIV therapy regimens. *Patient Educ Couns*, 50, pp. 187–199.

Space L. (1981). The computer as psychometrician. *Behav Res Meth Instr*, 13, pp. 595.

Stevens-Simon C, Dolgan JI, Kelly L, *et al.* (1997). The effect of monetary incentives and peer support groups on repeat adolescent pregnancies: A randomized trial of the Dollar-a-Day Program. *JAMA*, 277, pp. 977–982.

Strasburger VC. (2006). Is there an unconscious conspiracy against teenagers in the United States? *Clin Pediatr*, 45, pp. 714–717.

Tideman RL, Chen MY, Pitts MK, Ginige S, Slaney M, Fairley CK. (2007). A randomised controlled trial comparing computer-assisted with face-to-face sexual history taking in a clinical setting. *Sex Transm Infect*, 83, pp. 52–56.

Tidwell J. (1998). House Calls of the Future. *Modern Maturity*, 41R, p. 8.

Timpka T, Graspemo G, Hassling L, Nordfeldt S, Eriksson H. (2004). Towards integration of computer games in interactive health education environments: understanding gameplay challenge, narrative and spectacle. *Stud Health Technol Inform*, 107, pp. 941–945.

Webb PM, Zimet GD, Fortenberry JD, Blythe MJ. (1999). Comparability of a computer-assisted versus written method for collecting health behavior information from adolescent patients. *J Adolesc Health*, 24, pp. 383–388.

Zurhellen WM. (1995). The computerization of ambulatory pediatric practice. *Pediatrics*, 96, pp. 835–842.

Chapter 10

Health Promotion

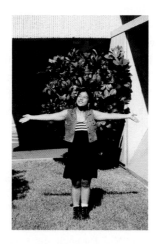

"When I need you to listen to me, and you start giving me advice or try to solve my problems, then you are part of them."

— 16-year-old

Health Guidance and Counseling

Interactive counseling allows both provider and youth to discuss beliefs, perceptions, options, and choices for health behaviors. The provider can help the youth accurately perceive and prioritize problems, come to agreement about how the solutions can solve problems, develop doable solutions, and create an implementation plan.

Reflective Listening Looks at Options to Solve Problems.

Steps in Exploring Options:

- Understand and be clear about the problem.
- "Brainstorm" alternatives (i.e. sexual behaviors).
- Evaluate various alternatives/possible outcomes.
- *Agree* on a solution.
- Avoid *shoulds*.
- Obtain a commitment, and plan a time for follow-up.

Promotion of healthy lifestyles and reduction of health risk behaviors helps youths make decisions to prevent disease, and develop long term positive health practices. Optimally, efforts are culturally and community-based, and include many others involved in the youth's life. Health information needs to be repeated and reinforced by many different sources. Many youths need to realize that they are vulnerable, but they also need practical knowledge and skills.

Questionnaires are useful for screening patients and their parents for health issues and health behaviors. The Brief Risk Screening Teen Questionnaire for patients (described in page 12) can be used together with the following Adolescent Health Questionnaire, often provided to a parent of a minor to complete.

Adolescent Health Questionnaire

This questionnaire is a way for us to most effectively address, share, and focus on all of the important health issues for the health evaluation today. Parent or patient, please circle "Yes" or "No" for each question.

1. Since the last visit, have there been any *major* illnesses or hospitalizations? .... No Yes
2. Taking any medication? .... No Yes
3. Ever had a bad fever reaction to a vaccine (> 104°F)? .... No Yes
4. Any concerns with skin rash? .... No Yes
5. Any concerns about weight? .... No Yes
6. Drinking low-fat or non-fat cow's milk? .... No Yes
7. Eating five servings of fruits and vegetables every day? .... No Yes
8. Eating breakfast every day? .... No Yes
9. Eat fast food more than once per week? .... No Yes
10. Using supplements such as creatine, andro, or steroids? .... No Yes

11. In the past year, any use of laxatives or diet pills, or self-induced vomiting to lose weight? .... No Yes
12. Any concerns about bowel movements or urinating? .... No Yes
13. Are teeth brushed every night? .... No Yes
14. Been to the dentist in the last year? .... No Yes
15. Any concerns with hearing or vision? .... No Yes
16. Ever been a victim of abuse, violence or molestation? .... No Yes
17. Any broken bones or bad injuries since last physical examination?
    .... No Yes
18. Getting 30 minutes or more of strenuous exercise four times per week?
    .... No Yes
19. Any difficulty with breathing during exercise? .... No Yes
20. Watching TV or doing video or computer or Internet more than 2 hours per day? .... No Yes
21. Had a discussion about TV, computer programs and Internet regarding sex and violence? .... No Yes
22. Is there a TV in the bedroom? .... No Yes
23. Being treated by a chiropractor, acupuncturist or using any homeopathic remedies? .... No Yes
24. Always wearing a helmet when riding a bike, skateboarding, roller-blading or riding a scooter? .... No Yes
25. Can swim well in deep water? .... No Yes
26. Any guns in your home, or ever carry any weapons? .... No Yes
27. Put on sunscreen when going out in the sun? .... No Yes
28. Ever been arrested, been in trouble with the law, or been in a gang?
    .... No Yes

Young women only:

1. Are periods irregular, longer than 7 days, or associated with real bad cramps?
   .... No Yes
2. Taking a multivitamin with iron every day? .... No Yes
3. Eating/drinking four servings of calcium foods daily, or taking a calcium pill? .... No Yes

Changing Youths' Health Behaviors

Do not hesitate to target specific issues or behaviors. Professionals tend to be too diffuse in our theoretical thinking.

Three Considerations Which Can be Approached Individually

1. Prevention vs Delay (e.g. sexual activity)
2. Non-use vs Responsible use (e.g. alcohol)
3. Potential risks of interventions (e.g. weight control)

Based on major health issues for adolescents, which can be reduced to single achievable behavior goals, there are six issues which have been identified.

Six Major Health Issues for Adolescents

- Intentional and unintentional injury
- Drug and alcohol use
- Sexual behavior (HIV, STD, pregnancy)
- Tobacco use
- Dietary behavior
- Physical activity

The following specifies six specific attainable behavioral goals, but several important areas are missing from these six priority behaviors. The missing issues are of great concern for mortality such as suicide, homicide, violence, firearms, and teen pregnancy, but they cannot be reduced to a single achievable behavior goal.

Six Achievable Adolescent Behavior Goals (to enhance longevity and health)

- Use seat belts.
- Do not drink (or use drugs) and drive.
- If you have sex, use condoms.
- Do not smoke.
- Eat a low-fat diet.
- Get regular aerobic exercise.

Healthy lifestyles and behaviors require knowledge (information, skills, attitudes, and beliefs), resources (supplies, helpers, easy access to services), and motivation (advocates, incentives and perceivable personal benefits, and peer approval). If a youth is to use a condom, there must be knowledge (why it is important to use one, how to do so effectively), resources (a condom), and motivation (partner approval and encouragement, desire for protection).

Essential Triad for Behavior Change

1. Knowledge: information, skills, beliefs
2. Resources: equipment, supplies, alternatives, access to health care
3. Motivation: positive incentives, peer approval, social sanctions

If the provider helps channel the motives, priorities and goals of a youth, then health promotion will succeed.

Culturally-Specific Health Education

The health risk behaviors of adolescents are nearly universal and cross-cultural worldwide. However, cultural differences among youths influence their perceptions about health and healthy behaviors. Providers must realize how their own health beliefs may differ from those of a youth, and that many of these beliefs are determined by ethnic, cultural, educational or economic factors. Community influences can also impact a youth's expectations about the consequences of certain health risk behaviors (i.e. drinking beer or wine is common and harmless). Not considering the culture of a youth can cause failure to correctly assess a problem, lack of cooperation, inadequate utilization of resources, or alienation of the youth.

Cultural factors affect a youth's health practices in many ways. Cultural beliefs about life, health, and illness may influence how a problem is understood. These beliefs and values can also influence perception of health information and education, as well as willingness to comply with advice. A youth may fail to discuss or disclose important information because of cultural beliefs about what problems require help, or what problems can even be discussed. Self-disclosure is sometimes a delicate matter, even further complicated by language barriers. Ethnic stereotypes and assumptions based on race or culture obstruct effective health guidance and the interactive opportunities. Guidance delivered by a provider in a culturally sensitive fashion will not only show respect for youths but also maximize the opportunity to establish a relationship that facilitates successful outcomes.

A provider needs both sensitivity and cultural knowledge, should offer respectful advice, and must become aware of *personal* cultural biases, orientations and experiences. For many cultural groups, parents and family play a very active role in decisions about health, and providers must understand these groups in order to be effective in developing realistic goals and facilitate compliance with advice and recommendations.

Changing Behavior and Life Skills

Changing behavior involves both *cognitive learning* and *social learning*. Cognitive learning includes the youth's attitudes, beliefs and self-efficacy that cause behavior change. Social learning involves attitudes and perceptions of social norms which are shaped by the attitudes and behaviors of role models in the social environment, and the youth's involvement with peer role models. Good decision making requires tools such as *assertiveness* techniques, which is meeting one's own needs while being sensitive to the needs of others. This is a skill which takes practice, but can be a positive preventive tool which enables win-win solutions and pre-empts conflicts.

Additional Life Skills Needed for Success and Well-being

- Decision making skills and commitment.
- Problem solving.
- Coping skills.
- Stress management.
- Conflict resolution and anger management.
- Resisting peer pressure.
- Communication and interpersonal relationship skills.
- Seeking out reliable support and resources.

Principles of Adolescent Education and Counseling

- Screen all adolescents.
- Develop a therapeutic alliance.
- Ensure that adolescents understand the relationship between behavior and health.
- Work with adolescents to assess barriers to behavior change.
- Involve patients in selecting risk factors to change.
- Use a combination of strategies.
- Design a behavior modification plan.
- Gain commitment from adolescents to change.
- Monitor progress through follow-up contact.
- Involve office staff, paraprofessionals, and use peer counselors.

Prochaska's Stages of Readiness to Change

The widely used transtheoretical model of Prochaska and DiClemente describes several stages through which people normally pass in the process of changing. Staged Behavior Change models [Prochaska, 1992] help the provider identify the position of the youth in terms of *readiness to change*. Six stages are discussed below, and the provider will obtain optimal results if he/she can direct motivation to change behavior *to the stage of readiness to change* of the youth, and design interventions based on that stage, as well as the developmental stage.

Precontemplation is the state in which people are not considering change. People tend to leave this stage permanently once they begin to contemplate.

Contemplation is the stage characterized by ambivalence or a more conscious decisional balance process. "Confronting" contemplators is likely to evoke resistance by eliciting counter argument. Prochaska and DiClemente have at times distinguished between early and late contemplators, depending on the extent to which they are experimenting with approaching change.

Decision or *determination* was a stage included in the original transtheoretical model. It implies a moment or window of opportunity in which the person has made a firm decision or commitment to change but may not yet have taken action. Depending on who you talk to, some people still consider this a part of the model, others no not.

Action is the stage characterized by the taking of action in order to achieve change. It persists as long as active change efforts are underway and the change goal has not been attained.

Maintenance is the stage where once a change goal has been attained, the challenge is to prevent backsliding or relapse. Efforts to maintain change often involve different strategies from those used to achieve change in the first place.

Relapse is sometimes described as a separate stage occurring when the person's maintenance efforts have failed, and sometimes the event of relapse is seen simply as movement from Maintenance back into Precontemplation or Contemplation.

Brief Negotiation

Brief Negotiation is a collaborative, patient-centered method for increasing an adolescent's motivation to consider health behavior change and to negotiate the best course of action, in brief clinical encounters.

Process

The health provider does not assume an authoritarian role and attempts to draw on and enhance patients' internal motivation to make health behavior changes based on their own decisions and choices. The focus shifts from giving information, advice, and behavior change prescriptions to helping patients explore concerns, ambivalence, reasons for change, and ideas and strategies for change. The health provider utilizes a variety of negotiating strategies based on a patient's readiness to consider change. A patient's readiness to change can be understood by Prochaska's Stages of Change. There is a fundamental belief that the capacity and potential for making behavior change is in every one of us.

Goals

Goals of Brief Negotiation

1. To establish rapport by using an empathetic, non-judgmental style.
2. Emphasize patients' freedom of choice to make decisions regarding their health.

3. Understand and accept the adolescent's feelings and thoughts about the health condition and/or health behavior change issue.
4. Collaborate with the adolescent to explore motivation and confidence about health behavior change.
5. Create an environment that encourages the adolescent to think and speak about the concerns, ambivalence, reasons for change, and ideas and strategies for health behavior change.
6. Individualize the negotiating strategies based on the adolescent's readiness to consider change.
7. Minimize resistance by not confronting, pushing, or persuading.
8. Enhance the adolescent's self-confidence by expressing your confidence in their ability to change when ready.

Style

Key Elements of Brief Negotiation Style

1. Understanding: Empathetic, careful listening, attentive, non-judgmental, warm, and supportive. Seeking to see things from the adolescent's perspective.
2. Patient-centered: Encourage the adolescent to be as active as possible in making decisions about needed health behavior change. Eliciting motivation to change from the adolescent, not imposing it from without. Encouraging the adolescent to do most of the talking.
3. Collaborative: Pursuing common goals, sharing of agendas and responsibility, working together in partnership to determine the best course of action.
4. Individualized: Tailoring intervention approaches to match the adolescent's personal needs and readiness to change, moving at the adolescent's pace.
5. Emphasizing freedom of choice: Acknowledging that the decision if, when, and how to change is the adolescent's. Avoiding "restrictive" messages (e.g. "you must", or "you can't").
6. Respectful/Accepting: Conveying respect by accepting whatever decisions an adolescent makes about health behavior change.

Elements

Studies of brief intervention identify common effective elements of effective counseling [Bien, 1993]. They found six components present in all or most effective brief interventions, represented by the acronym FRAMES.

Elements of Effective Brief Intervention: FRAMES

- Feedback: Effective brief interventions often provide clients with personal feedback regarding their individual status. This can include confirmation of problems associated with the behavior (i.e. the relationship between smoking and asthma), feedback on personal behavior relative to norms (i.e. comparison of how much the person reports drinking with the average for similar people), information about laboratory or other assessed values, etc. Such feedback is not to be confused with giving people information about the problem behavior in general.
- Responsibility: Effective brief interventions have also emphasized the individual's freedom of choice and personal responsibility for change. General themes are: 1. It's up to you; you're free to decide to change or not; 2. No one else can decide for you or force you to change; 3. You're the one who has to do it if it's going to happen.
- Advice: Nevertheless, effective brief counseling has almost universally included a clear recommendation or advice on the need for change, typically in a supportive and concerned, rather than authoritarian, manner.
- Menu: When specific strategies for change have been offered, they have often been in menu form — providing a variety of options from among which clients may pick those that seem more suitable or appealing.
- Empathy: When provider style has been described in studies of effective brief intervention, emphasis has been placed on an empathic, reflective, warm, and supportive manner.
- Self-efficacy: Finally, effective brief interventions have also often reinforced the client's expectation that he or she *can* change.

A more detailed discussion of FRAMES elements can be found in a number of books on motivational interviewing [Fuller, 2008; Rollnick, Miller, Butler, 2007]. It is also a noteworthy aspect that most studies of effective brief intervention have included ongoing follow-up contacts, which may themselves reinforce change even if conducted solely for research purposes. Some studies have shown that follow-up interviews in themselves promote change.

Suggested Readings and Bibliography

Anderson LM, Scrimshaw SC, Fullilove MT, Fielding JE, Normand J; Task Force on Community Preventive Services. (2003). Culturally competent healthcare systems. A systematic review. *Am J Prev Med*, 24 (Suppl 3), pp. 68–79.

Bartlett EE. (1984). Effective approaches to patient education for the busy pediatrician. *Pediatrics*, 74 (Suppl), pp. 920–923.

Berg-Smith SM, Stevens VJ, Brown KM, *et al.* (1999). A brief motivational intervention to improve dietary adherence in adolescents. *Health Educ Res*, 14, pp. 399–410.

Bien TH, Miller WR, Tonigan JS. (1993). Brief interventions for alcohol problems: a review. *Addiction*, 88, pp. 315–335.

Contreras B, Ewan C. (1996). A culturally-specific oral health program for high risk Vietnamese children. *Probe*, 30, pp. 156–157.

DiClemente RJ, Wingood GM, Crosby RA, *et al.* (2001). A prospective study of psychological distress and sexual risk behavior among black adolescent females. *Pediatrics*, 108, p. E85.

Ferguson SL. (1998). Peer counseling in a culturally specific adolescent pregnancy prevention program. *J Health Care Poor Underserved*, 9, pp. 322–340.

Fuller C. (2008). *A Toolkit of Motivational Skills: Encouraging and Supporting Change in Individuals*. 2nd Edn. (Wiley, USA).

Herek GM, Gillis JR, Glunt EK, Lowis J, Welton D, Capitanio JP. (1998). Culturally sensitive AIDS educational videos for African American audiences: effects of source, message, receiver, and context. *Am J Community Psychol*, 26, pp. 705–743.

Joffe A, Radius S, Gall M. (1988). Health counseling for adolescents: what they want, what they get, and who gives it. *Pediatrics*, 82, pp. 481–485.

Molyneux J. (2007). Cost-effective, culturally specific diabetes care. *Am J Nurs*, 107, p. 20.

Prochaska JO, DiClemente CC, Norcross JC. (1992). In search of how people change. Applications to addictive behaviors. *Am Psychol,* 47, pp. 1102–1114.

Rollnick S, Miller W, Butler C. (2007). *Motivational Interviewing in Health Care: Helping Patients Change Behavior (Applications of Motivational Interviewing)*. (The Guilford Press, New York).

Rotheram-Borus MJ, Piacentini J, Miller S, Graae F, Castro-Blanco D. (1994). Brief cognitive-behavioral treatment for adolescent suicide attempters and their families. *J Am Acad Child Adolesc Psychiatry*, 33, pp. 508–517.

Runkle C, Osterholm A, Hoban R, McAdam E, Tull R. (2000). Brief negotiation program for promoting behavior change: the Kaiser Permanente approach to continuing professional development. *Educ Health (Abingdon)*, 13, pp. 377–386.

Tyler DO, Horner SD. (2008). Family-centered collaborative negotiation: a model for facilitating behavior change in primary care. *J Am Acad Nurse Pract*, 20, pp. 194–203.

Welch SJ, Holborn SW. (1988). Contingency contracting with delinquents: effects of a brief training manual on staff contract negotiation and writing skills. *J Appl Behav Anal*, 21, pp. 357–368.

Wilson SR, Strub P, Buist AS, *et al.* (2010). Shared treatment decision making improves adherence and outcomes in poorly controlled asthma. *Am J Respir Crit Care Med*, 181, pp. 566–577.

Suggested Websites

Student Counseling Virtual Pamphlet Collection is sponsored by the University of Chicago Student Counseling and Resource Service. This site brings together online pamphlets emanating from a number of different universities. Topics covered include alcohol, anger, anxiety, cults, depression, suicide, homesickness, and counseling, among others: http://counseling.uchicago.edu/vpc/virtulets.html

Healthfinder: http://www.healthfinder.gov

TeensHealth, sponsored by the Nemours Foundation, is a site which provides teens with a wide range of online health, mental health, and social information. Topics include nutrition, drugs, STDs, contraception, sports, homework, baby sitting, volunteering, stress management, and safety, among others: http://kidshealth.org/teen

Internet Public Library - Teen Division (Health) - is under the aegis of the School of Information and Library Studies at the University of Michigan. It is a consumer site for a wide variety of health information resources. This URL is the page for teens and young adults with links to site relating to body image and eating disorders, diseases, exercise, hygiene, mental health, nutrition, puberty, sex, and substance abuse: http://www.ipl.org/cgi-bin/teen/teen.db.out.pl?id-he000

Tips 4 Teens (Centers for Disease Control) is a site which provides resources for adolescents and young adults about a variety of topics: http://www.cdc.gov/HealthyYouth/az/index.htm

Youth Health Program Software

©2010 HealthMedia Corporation — www.HealthMediaCorp.com
(reprinted with permission)

Assessment questions, with three approximate levels of branching designated by two indentations (complex branching algorithms not shown; comprehensive Medical and Sports evaluation questions excluded)

Are you Male or Female?
Which describes you best? [Race]
    Which of one these do you relate to most?

Hello! I am your confidential Youth Health Provider computer, and I will be asking you about you and your health. At the end, I will give you some very helpful advice and ideas on things you should know about yourself, and on things you should check on with a Health Provider, such as a doctor, a nurse, or other health worker.
Type your FIRST NAME or NICKNAME.
Very good, [NAME]. I will be asking you questions, and they are private. You'll get a lot of very helpful information back about yourself when we're done, but I need you to give me true answers about yourself so I can give you the right results.
By the way, [NAME], think about each question very carefully. If you make a mistake, you can back up a few questions to correct your answers by pressing the Tab key, but once you've finished, you can't go back to change your answers. Some of the questions will seem very personal. That's OK, nobody should be watching you.

Now, please give your birthdate. Type the Month-Day-Year LIKE THIS: 6-22-2010.

Who do you now live with?

Do you have your own health provider or doctor that you can easily talk to alone about private matters?

Please type the biggest worries or health concerns that you would like to ask or talk about with a health provider. Use only one line across the screen, or you can type NONE.

Have you had a health checkup by a health provider in the last 3 years?

Have you been to a dentist in the last 2 years?

Do you brush your teeth at bedtime every night?

How many times a week do you do exercise or sports (that make you sweat or breathe hard) for more than a half hour without stopping?

Are you now taking any medicines (like pills or syrup) that a health provider gave you?

Have you recently taken any medicines that were bought at the store or market (over-the-counter medicines)?

Very good [NAME]. How do you feel your weight is, now?

Do you sometimes drive a car, truck, or van?

Have you driven around at fast speeds with friends in the past 3 months?

When you drive or ride in a car, truck, or van, how often do you wear a seat belt?

> When you ride in a car, truck, or van, how often do you wear a seat belt?

Do you sometimes rollerblade, skateboard, or ride a bicycle?

> How often do you wear a helmet when you rollerblade, skateboard, or ride a bicycle?

Do you sometimes ride a motorcycle, minibike, or all-terrain vehicle (ATV)?

> How often do you wear a helmet when you ride a motorcycle, minibike, or all-terrain vehicle (ATV)?

Is there a gun, BB-gun, or other firearm in your home, or where you live?

During the last 12 months, did you use a handgun, rifle, BB-gun, or shotgun for any reason, including hunting or target shooting?

You've done very well, [NAME]. The next questions are very important.

Are you having problems with learning at school or with your progress in classes?

Do you have a paying job now?

> Do you have a pretty good idea of what you want to do for your career or future work?

Has there ever been a time when you smoked more than one cigarette every day?

In the last 30 days, how often did you smoke cigarettes?

In the last 7 days, how often did you smoke cigarettes?

Have you ever used chewing tobacco, snuff, dip, or smokeless tobacco?

In the last 30 days, how often did you use chewing tobacco, snuff, dip, or smokeless tobacco?

Alcohol includes beer, wine and other booze. Did you ever drink alcohol and then drive a car, truck, van, motorcycle, or boat?

In the last 3 months, did you drink alcohol and then drive a car, truck, van, motorcycle, or boat?

In the last 30 days, how often did you drink any kind of beer, wine, or other alcoholic drinks?

In the last 30 days, when you drank, about how many drinks did you usually have each time?

Have you ever had enough alcoholic drinks to get drunk, pass out, or black out?
Has anyone ever given you a hard time, or have you been in trouble because of drinking alcohol?

Have you ever felt you ought to cut down on your drinking?
Have people annoyed you by criticizing your drinking?
Have you ever felt bad or guilty about your drinking?
Have you ever had a drink first thing in the morning to steady your nerves or get rid of a hangover?
Do you feel drinking helps you relax?
Do you feel drinking helps you be friendly?
Do you feel drinking helps you be with friends who drink?
Do you feel drinking helps you forget problems?
Do you feel drinking helps you feel good about yourself?

How often have you been a rider in a car, truck or van when the driver had been drinking alcohol or using drugs?
Have you done it in the last 6 months?

In the last 6 months, how often did you drive a car, truck, van, or boat after drinking alcohol or using drugs that get you high or loaded?

Many drugs can be bought at the store or market without seeing a doctor. How often have you used such drugs to get to sleep, stay awake, calm down, or get high?
Marijuana products include weed, dope, grass, pot, buds, hash, oil, and Thai stick. Have you used any of these in the last 6 months?

How often have you used marijuana products in the last 3 months?

How often have you used marijuana products in the last 1 month?

Do you sometimes smoke marijuana and drink alcohol together?

Have you ever used any kind of drugs such as cocaine, crack, angel dust, LSD, acid, MDA, ecstasy, speed, ice, heroin, or narcotics?
Have you ever used any medicine to get loaded or high, such as uppers, downers, or other pills, when you didn't need them for a health problem?

Have you ever used cocaine, crack, freebase, or rock?

Have you used cocaine or crack in the last 6 months?
How often have you used it in the last 3 months?
Do you sometimes feel a need or desire for it?
How often have you used it in the last 30 days?

Have you ever used speed, crystal meth, ice, dexies, amphetamines, uppers, stimulants? (This doesn't include stay-awake or diet pills from a store or market.)

Have you used speed, crystal meth or ice in the last 6 months?
How often have you used it in the last 3 months?
Do you sometimes feel a need or desire for it?
How often have you used it in the last 30 days?

Have you ever used heroin, smack, percodan, morphine, or narcotic pain pills?

Have you used narcotics or smack in the last 6 months?
How often have you used it in the last 3 months?
Do you sometimes feel a need or desire for it?
How often have you used it in the last 30 days?

Have you ever used drugs like LSD, acid, magic mushrooms, MDA, X or ecstasy?

How often have you used drugs like acid, mushrooms, or ecstasy in the last 3 months?
How often have you used it in the last 30 days?
Have you ever used PCP, angel dust, or hog?
How often have you used PCP or angel dust in the last 3 months?
How often have you used it in the last 30 days?

Have you ever used downers, barbiturates, reds, yellows, valium, ludes, or tranquilizers (without a doctor telling you to)?

How often have you used downers or tranquilizers in the last 3 months?
How often have you used it in the last 30 days?

In the last 3 months, how often have you taken any of those drugs along with alcoholic drinks?
Have you ever shot up or injected drugs into yourself with a needle?
Have you ever taken insulin shots?

Have you ever sniffed glue, breathed in spray cans, or inhaled other solvents or gas to get high?

How often have you sniffed glue or inhaled sprays or gasses in the last 3 months?

Have you ever used steroids ("roids" or "juice") for sports training or muscle building?

Have you used steroids in the last 3 months?

Now I'd like to ask you how you feel about things, [NAME].
Are you often nervous or tense, or do you have a lot of worries, pressure or stress?
Do you have problems at home with your parents or family?
Did you have problems at home with your parents or family?
A physical fight is when people hit, kick, punch or attack each other. It's not when there is only yelling or shouting. Has there been physical fighting in your home?

During the last 6 months, how often did you see or were you involved in a physical family fight, where someone could have been or was hurt?

In the past 3 months, has an adult in your family, or an adult you live with, badly injured you or beat you up on purpose?
Have you ever ran away from home overnight or longer?
Do you often argue or get in trouble with friends, parents or other people because they don't understand you?
Do you often get mad, lose your temper, or have fights with friends, parents or others?
To protect yourself, have you ever carried a weapon like a gun, knife, razor, ice pick, pipe, bat or club?

Have you carried a weapon in the last 3 months?
Have you ever carried a gun to protect yourself?

Have you carried a gun in the last 3 months?

Thanks, [NAME]. Are you mostly happy with the way things are going for you these days?

During the past 3 months, have you often been sad or unhappy?

During the past 4 weeks have you often felt hopeless?

Have you been to a counselor for help with your problems?

During the past 4 weeks, how often have you felt really down, or like you have nothing to look forward to?

You know, [NAME], when some people get very sad or upset, they think about killing themselves. Did you ever seriously think about doing that?

> Did you ever make a plan to kill yourself?
>
> [NAME], did you ever try to kill yourself, or hurt yourself in a way that you could die?
>
> In the last 3 months, how often did you think about killing yourself?
>
> > In the last 4 weeks, how often did you think about killing yourself?

Is there anyone in your close family who tried to, or did, kill himself or herself on purpose?

Did you have a friend who killed himself or herself on purpose?

Is there an adult you can easily talk to about your problems?

> Is there an adult you would turn to for help if you were really upset?
>
> > Is there someone you would turn to for help if you were really upset?

[NAME], THANK YOU for being so honest. The last questions are about private things, but they are very important. You'll want to give true answers, and when we're done, the results I'll give you will be helpful for you.

Do you have any children of your own?

> Would you like to have a baby and become a parent now, rather than wait till later in your life?
>
> > Would you like to have another baby now, rather than wait till later in your life?

Would you like to learn more about birth control and how to not get pregnant?

Does it burn or hurt when you urinate or pee lately?

Have you recently had a drip, discharge, or pus coming from your penis? (M = Males)

Lately, have you had anything smelly or strange, like pus, coming from your vagina?

Have you ever had a menstrual period (a monthly blood flow)?

Sexually-transmitted disease is called STD or VD, and it's spread by sexual contact. Some are gonorrhea, chlamydia, syphilis, genital herpes, genital warts, HIV and AIDS. Would you like to learn more about how not to get STDs?

Have you ever been told by a health provider that you had a sexually-transmitted disease?

Has anyone ever touched your sex organs or other private parts, when you didn't want them to?

Has anyone ever tried to force you to have sex when you didn't want to?

Has anyone ever forced you to have sex with them?

    Has this happened in the last 6 months?

Do you mostly feel more sexually attracted to females than males? M

    Do you mostly feel more sexually attracted to males than females? M

Do you worry about being sexually attracted to other males? M

Do you mostly feel more sexually attracted to males than females?

    Do you mostly feel more sexually attracted to females than males?

Do you worry about being sexually attracted to other females?

Have you ever used any kind of birth control? (besides not having sex)

Have you ever been pregnant?

Do you have a boyfriend now?

Have you ever gotten someone pregnant? M

Do you have a girlfriend now? M

Have you ever had oral sex, where your mouth touched someone's sex organs, or where someone's mouth touched your sex organs?

Sexual intercourse is when the penis (the male sex organ) is put inside the vagina (the female sex organ). Have you ever had sexual intercourse? (What I mean is, have you have put your penis into a vagina?) M

Sexual intercourse is when the penis (the male sex organ) is put inside the vagina (the female sex organ). Have you ever had sexual intercourse? (What I mean is, has a penis has been put inside your vagina?)

Some of your answers about sex don't fit with each other. Let's go back and try again.

    In your lifetime, have you had sex contacts with more than one male?

    Have you had a sexually-transmitted disease checkup or been to a STD clinic in the last 6 months?

    The last time you had sexual intercourse, did you two use a condom?

    Have you had sexual intercourse (in the vagina) during the last 6 months?

        During the past 6 months, how many different people did you have sexual intercourse with?

        In your whole life, how many different people have you had sexual contact or intercourse with?

    When you have had sex, how often did you or your partner use some kind of birth control?

When you had sexual intercourse in the last 6 months, did you use a condom every time? M

When you had sexual intercourse in the last 6 months, did your partner use a condom every time?

Did you use a female vaginal condom every time?
Do you have Norplant (a birth control implant) in your arm right now?
Have you ever had the Depo-Provera birth control shot?

What was the date of your last Depo-Provera shot? (If you're not exactly sure, enter your closest guess.) Type the Month-Day-Year LIKE THIS: 1-14-2010.

The last time you had sexual intercourse, what did you or your partner do or use to prevent pregnancy?
Do you feel that birth control pills are not safe?

Do you feel that birth control shots are not safe?
Would you like your girlfriend to get pregnant in the next few months? M
Would you like to get someone pregnant in the next few months? M

Have you had a checkup by a health provider for VD or sexually-transmitted disease in the last year?
Have you had a checkup by a health provider for VD or sexually-transmitted disease since the last time you had sex?
Have you ever had a pap test or pelvic exam, where a health provider looks in your vagina and checks your uterus?

Please enter the date (month-year) of your last pelvic exam, LIKE THIS: 4-2010.
Would you like to get pregnant in the next few months?
Do you wonder if you have something wrong with you so you can't get pregnant?

Do your menstrual periods mostly come on time?
Normally, how many days are there between your menstrual periods? Type the 2 digit number LIKE THIS: 28.
Have you had a menstrual period in the last 3 months?
When was your last menstrual period? (The FIRST day it started) Type the Month-Day-Year LIKE THIS: 2-13-2010.

Would you say your period is late for you at this time?
Have you had sexual intercourse since your last menstrual period?
Are you currently having sexual intercourse more often than once every 2 weeks or so?

Do you now have a positive pregnancy test?

Was it done by a health provider, hospital or clinic?
Was it done at home or by a self-test kit?
When was it done? Type the month-year LIKE THIS: 4-2010.

Have you been told by a health provider or clinic that you are pregnant at this time?

Have you been to a doctor or health provider to check this pregnancy yet?

Have you ever had blood clots in your legs?

THANK YOU, [NAME]. You have done very well.
Please tell me how honest you were when answering these questions. (scale 1–5)
You don't have to give your printout to a health provider, but it's important that he or she knows about everything that can affect your health, so he or she can do their best to help you. Unless it's not safe or it's an emergency, your health provider will keep your answers private.

Would you please allow me to let your health provider know about your sexual abuse?
Would you please allow me to let your health provider know about you carrying a gun?

VERY GOOD. Your results have been computed. Your *personalized health presentation* will soon begin.
When I'm done printing, carefully remove the paper. It was great talking with you! PLEASE share your paper with a health provider. Thank you for working with me, [NAME].
…then find the numbers at the bottom for the HANDOUTS.
Before you leave the room, take a handout for each number printed at the bottom.

Handout and Video Library Subjects (prioritized order of presentations)

Key: Preprinted handouts by gender (Both, Male, Female, * = not preprintable; printed by computer) ~ Topic ~ Reviewers

Health Risk Problems Identified

B ~ Suicide and Depression ~ Elster, Sahler, Ning, Collins
MF ~ Abstinc, Sex, Birth Control ~ Elster, Neinstein, Ning, Collins
B ~ Male Condom Use ~ Elster, Neinstein, Ning, Collins
* ~ Driving Under the Influence ~ Elster, Hammar, Ning, Collins

B ~ Carrying Guns and Weapons ~ Elster, Hammar, Ning, Collins
B ~ Drug Abuse/Prevention ~ Elster, Farrow, Ning, Collins
B ~ Substance Abuse of Cocaine and Crack ~ Farrow, Ning, Collins
B ~ Substance Abuse of Solvents ~ Farrow, Ning, Collins
B ~ Substance Abuse of Stimulants ~ Farrow, Ning, Collins
B ~ Substance Abuse of Narcotics and Opiates ~ Farrow, Ning, Collins
B ~ Substance Abuse of Hallucinogens ~ Farrow, Ning, Collins
B ~ Substance Abuse of Tranquilizers and Sedatives ~ Farrow, Ning, Collins
B ~ Sexual Abuse ~ Hammar, Ning, Collins
B ~ AIDS Counseling/HIV Testing ~ Neinstein, Ning, Collins
* ~ Physical and Emotional Abuse ~ Hammar, Ning, Collins
* ~ Preventing Sexual Exploitation/Runaway ~ Farrow, Ning, Collins
MF ~ Sexual Orientation ~ Bidwell, Ning, Collins
F ~ Pregnancy and Concurrent Use of Drugs and Alcohol ~ Starn, Ning, Collins
F ~ Pregnancy and Early Prenatal Care ~ Starn, Ning, Collins
* ~ When Your Period is Late ~ Neinstein, Ning, Collins
MF ~ Desire for a Baby Now ~ Sahler, Ning, Collins
* ~ Anabolic Steroid Use ~ Farrow, Ning, Collins
B ~ Substance Abuse of Alcohol ~ Farrow, Ning, Collins
B ~ Substance Abuse of Marijuana ~ Farrow, Ning, Collins
* ~ Sexual Intercourse with Alcohol and Drugs ~ Neinstein, Ning, Collins
* ~ Erroneous Infertility Belief ~ Neinstein, Ning, Collins
B ~ STDs/(F) Pelvic Exam ~ Neinstein, Ning, Collins
* ~ Seat Belt Use ~ Ning, Collins
* ~ Bicycle Safety and Helmet Use ~ Ning, Collins
* ~ Guns at Home/Safety ~ Bidwell, Ning, Collins
* ~ Anorexia and Eating Disorders ~ Sahler, Hammar, Ning, Collins
B ~ Smoking/Tobacco Cessation ~ Farrow, Ning, Collins
B ~ Anger Management ~ Sahler, Ning, Collins
B ~ Communication Skills, Assertiveness Skills ~ Sahler, Ning, Collins
B ~ Conflict Resolution ~ Sahler, Ning, Collins
* ~ Concerns about Your Body ~ Ning, Collins
B ~ Getting Adequate Exercise; Fitness ~ Hammar, Ning, Collins
B ~ Overweight/Weight Management ~ Hammar, Ning, Collins
B ~ CHD Risk Factors/Cholesterol, Fat ~ Hammar, Ning, Collins
* ~ High Blood Pressure ~ Hammar, Ning, Collins
B ~ School Performance/Attendance, Career ~ Sahler, Ning, Collins
B ~ Stress Management Techniques ~ Sahler, Ning, Collins
B ~ Skin Cancer ~ Hammar, Ning, Collins

Anticipatory Guidance

MF ~ Relationships and Sex ~ Neinstein, Ning, Collins
B ~ Before Using Tobacco ~ Farrow, Ning, Collins
B ~ Personal Safety and Injury Reduction ~ Hammar, Ning, Collins
B ~ Puberty and Growing Up (M&F) ~ Hammar, Ning, Collins
F ~ Puberty and Growing Up (F only) ~ Hammar, Ning, Collins
M ~ Puberty and Growing Up (M only) ~ Hammar, Ning, Collins
* ~ Getting Health Care; School/Voc; Emotions/Depression ~ Bidwell, Ning, Collins
B ~ Eating Right/Weight Management ~ Miyasato, Nagata, Ning, Collins
* ~ The 6 Golden Rules for Youth Health ~ Ning, Collins
* ~ Dental Hygiene ~ Ning, Collins
B ~ Breast Self-Exam (F only) ~ Bidwell, Ning, Collins
B ~ Testicular Self-Exam (M only) ~ Bidwell, Ning, Collins

Educational Review Board

Arthur Elster MD — A.M.A., Department of Adolescent Health — Chicago, IL
Barry Collins PhD — UCLA Department of Psychology — Los Angeles, CA
James Farrow MD — University of Washington, Adolescent Clinic — Seattle, WA
Jane Starn RNC, DrPH — Pediatric Nurse Practitioner — Honolulu, HI
Larry Neinstein MD — Director, USC Student Health Center — Los Angeles, CA
Lily Ning MD — University of Hawaii, Student Health Service — Honolulu, HI
O.J. Sahler MD — Department of Education, AAP — Elk Grove Village, IL
Robert Bidwell MD — Kapiolani Children's Medical Center — Honolulu, HI
Sherrel L. Hammar MD — Kapiolani Children's Medical Center — Honolulu, HI

Index